Spasm

Living a Life With Cerebral Palsy

By Kerry Coe

SPASM

By Kerry Coe

ISBN: 9798552062522

Author Website:

www.spasm.org.uk

Twitter: @KerryCoe10

Illustrations by Kevan Thompson. A special thank you goes to Kev Thompson who has drawn all the illustrations for this book. For further details and private enquires for Kev's work please see details below:

Twitter: @KevanThompson2

Facebook: Kevan Thompson

"A life story about a young girl changing into a woman who has had to juggle many obstacles with cerebral palsy."

~ Dylan-Grace

Dear Sally

I can't believe it's 30 years since we last caught up.

Remember our schooldays? Such a laugh, always getting into trouble! The terrible two, that's what they used to call us.

Time goes so fast when you're enjoying yourself! You'll never guess what I've been up to since the age of 14.

I came fourth in The Best of British Youth, a national competition on Radio 4, when I was 14.

They sent me to Coventry (I sent myself really!) to college for four years to study to be a social worker. What a brilliant time!

- Had my first boyfriend
- Learnt to drive
- Starred in a Bafta Award winning film
- And loads more…

It was amazing but didn't stop there! I went to university and got my degree, who would have thought it? You know me, bloody-minded. If someone says, 'You can't do It,' I've always got to prove them wrong!

I moved on to independent living, or so I thought, and eventually fell in love and got married. There's lots, lots more - bits that made me chuckle, cry and scared me stiff.

Enjoy reading!

All my love now and always,

Kerry xx

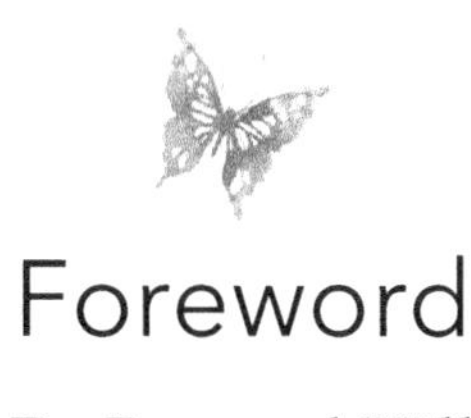

Foreword

By Bernard Hill

Kerry Noble and I met on the BBC Screen 2 film, Skallagrigg in 1993. I was playing her dad. My daughter in the film happened to be very assertive, bossy, confident and self-opinionated.

Kerry was very good casting.

I quickly got to know how she dealt with her world. "Don't call us handicapped. We're not handicapped. You're our handicap, you able-bodied people." "Having cerebral palsy defines the disability, not the person."

Each time we talked, I was taken up the learning ladder a little more. Each 'rung' was as surprising as the one before. Eventually, the whole Film Crew were led to the ladder, as it were.

The First Assistant Director runs the filming. Among many

other things that they do is call us all to arms, for a 'take'.

First take on Skallagrigg. We go to our start positions. Camera, lighting, sound, ready. A semi-silence falls on the set. First AD orders, "Stand by." It's a bit like "Take your marks!" in the 100 Metre Final.

It is not supposed to be followed by a voice from the other side of the set shouting, "I can't pukkin' stand!"

The silence, as the pennies dropped, was as long as a lifetime of ignorance.

"Who said that?" said the First, with a certain smile of appreciation. "Me. Kerry. How can I stand by?!"

After that, we all knew exactly who and where we were.

Kerry introduced me to new levels of insight into what it's like to be disabled; the real world the disabled live in and the terrible, unrepeatable jokes that disabled people tell about disabled people.

I learned how she brought her local Council to heel, in much the same way that she brought our film crew to heel, when she campaigned to have the doors changed on her local shopping arcade.

I came away from filming Skallagrigg with Kerry, a much wiser person. I felt I understood her world in a more intimate way.

I am now at ease in the company of disabled people. So I should be. It is harder for us, though. Disabled people are more used to dealing with able-bodied people. They manipulate us constantly in order to get what they want, what they need, to move around, to get on or off things.

What I learned from Kerry was how to accept that controversial truth. As far as able-bodied people being at a disadvantage, Kerry's attitude was, "Get over it. It's your fault and it's up to you to correct it." Hard words and tough lessons.

Apparently, I learned them well.

We were having our end of film party in a hotel. I was admiring the action on the dance floor; able-bodied and disabled jiving, break-dancing, wheelchair waltzes.

Ian Dury came and stood next to me and I told him how emotional I found it all.

He turned to me and said, "It's a secret society and you've just become a member."

I got there because Kerry Noble did that for me.

In this book, you will find moments and lessons. You may even find your own way to understanding what it is to be an ordinary human being, with a disability. If you do, welcome to the club.

About Me

Kerry Jane, that's my name
Passionate, determined and bloody minded
That's Kerry Jane
Full steam ahead
Nothing will stand in my way
That's Kerry Jane

Strong, determined, reliable
But never cross Kerry Jane
You only have one chance
So don't fuck it up!

Just a few words from me to you, a word of warning!

Don't read this if you're easily offended. Don't read this if you're politically correct. Don't read this if you don't like the truth. Don't read this if you're jealous.

I've written **MY** autobiography how **I** want to write it. I realise that I may have different viewpoints to other people involved with disabled people, but this is my account of my life so I use certain phrases in it, positive tense, and it's my humour and personality. I don't wish to impose my views on anybody. It's just how I see the world, and I strongly believe this is what has made me into the person I am today.

Throughout the book I refer to myself as a "**spastic**" and I feel it's extremely positive. It's my way of breaking down barriers and allowing people to feel at ease with my abnormal body movements and speech. I appreciate that not every disabled person shares the same humour **but** an autobiography is what it is! I apologise now if I offend people, it's how one person has survived a spastic body!

Relax, chill & enjoy!

Leap Into the Unknown

Flying high above the clouds
Up, up we go
Plane full of scared people
Going up, up, up

Not me!
I am full of joy, anticipation, freedom and excitement
Going up, up, up

Oh shit… someone's just opened the door….!
There's no way back
It's down all the bloody way
Have to wait my turn
And watch all the other guys plunge their way through the sky

They look nervous wrecks
Fear across their faces
But I am still on a high
Laughing and cheering all the way
Waiting for my turn

Seems like it will never come
Sitting so close to a guy
Who is in control of my destiny
For the next ten minutes

Am I mad, am I crazy, am I fearless?
No…I'm fooking petrified
But still I need a new electric wheelchair!

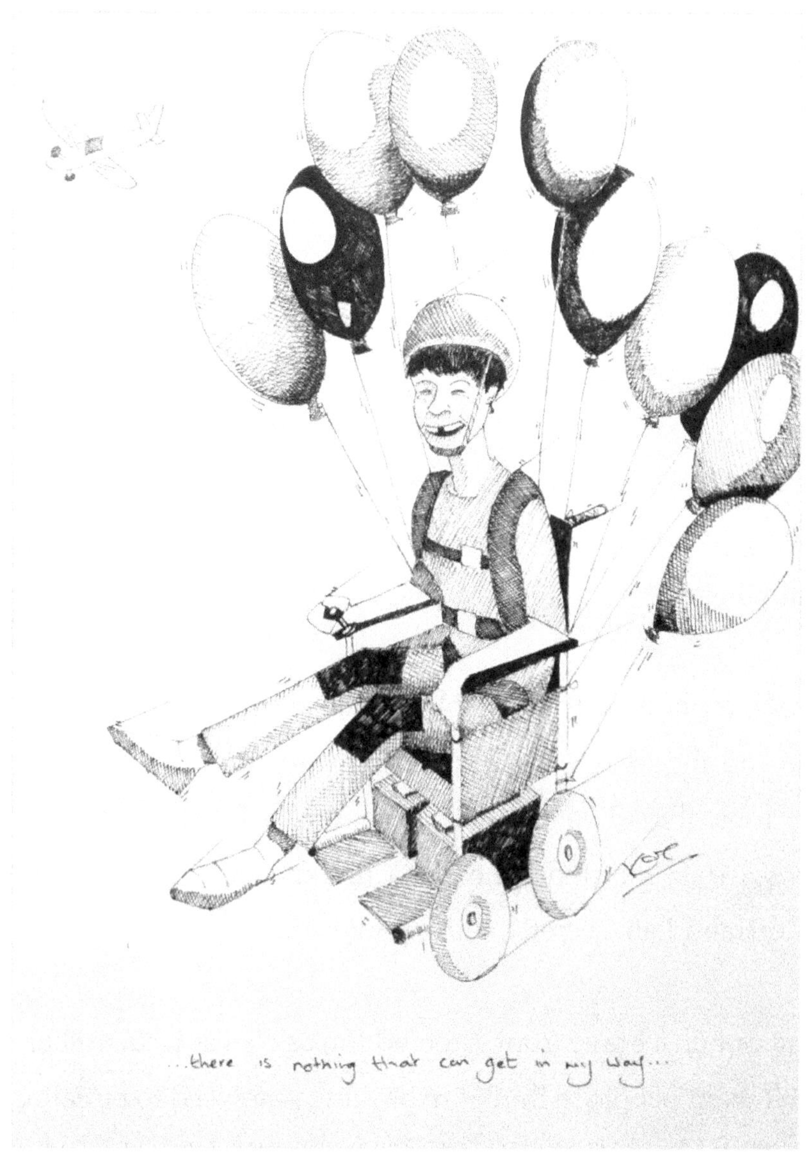
...there is nothing that can get in my way...

The Day Is Finally Here

Why the heck do I do this to myself? I spent last night wide awake, hoping for great weather.

Oh, my! Why me? Just a normal day, or is it? I've been waiting for this day for weeks, months, maybe years, and it's finally here!

I make a phone call to double/triple check I have the right date and the weather is OK. (I rung three times yesterday – they must think I've totally lost it but they do it three or four times a day, let alone once in a lifetime, so I'm sure they understand I am secretly shitting myself.)

Must put on a brave front, pretend I'm as cool as a cucumber. Don't want people to think I'm backing out. Need to be calm, collected, show the world 'Kerry can do this' (my life-long motto).

Where am I? Oh yeah, jumping out of a plane … yes, me!

Always been on my 'to do' list but never thought I would get the courage and enthusiasm to plunge 14,000 feet out of a bloody plane. And I'm *choosing* to do this?

I need to prove to myself and others I can meet this challenge head on (I always see challenges through, doesn't matter what it takes, tick it off my list). I was also raising money for my new 'hot wheels' with local people backing me.

I get ready as quickly as possible, not much time to think about the day ahead. Friends and family pick me up really early to take me to Langar Airfield. I put on a brave face and greet them with a huge smile. No act, honestly. I feel really at ease.

Travelling to the airfield seems to take forever and I chat all the way. Maybe nerves, or me being me? Don't know. Arriving an hour later my heart begins to race – this is really happening.

Determined to enjoy every second.

I meet the other 10 idiots I'm jumping with doing safety

training. No one says a bloody word. I inject some excitement and enthusiasm. There's not that much to remember for a tandem jump – cross your arms across your chest, lean back and smile for the camera! Easy.

Now for my biggest challenge – getting the bloody bright orange jumpsuit on! This takes two of us 10 to 15 minutes. Giggly and excited, can't control anything. Nerves getting the better of me?

Bell rings for my five-minute warning. Oh my God … oh shit … oh crap … what the heck, let's do this. That wheelchair will mean everything … Seems like forever getting on that bloody plane. There are 16 of us, including a cameraman, to prove I didn't chicken out. This is once-in-a-lifetime, or is it? I need memories to treasure.

Atmosphere so subdued. Beginning to feel scared, I ease the situation by laughing and joking. Don't know about the others, but it really helps me. That's until that enormous door opens and the cold air and wind rushes in!

Bloody freezing. Watching everybody going before me

makes me panic for the first time. Then I hear my instructor say: "Don't forget to smile for the camera." It's alright after that. We hitch forward to the open doors and gently ease our way out, with the cameraman holding on to the door to take pictures.

Surreal. Floating high in the sky, not a care in the world, taking every bit in. Then all of a sudden AHH! A sharp jerk and a quick tug and I guess the parachute was open ... it seemed the longest two or three minutes of my life, and I guess it was. Being able to be set free amongst the clouds, forgetting about my CP, just me and my instructor floating around in the sky, amazing! I felt like a butterfly in the sky... Absolutely fantastic, words can't describe it. On cloud nine! Takes my breath away for the first few minutes, but I'm free and liberated. Feel like I want to burn my bra. The instructor lets me steer the parachute for a few minutes before letting it open and floating down to Earth.

Amazing, freezing, wonderful, free ... like a bird looking at a world so far below. Looks like a model village ... buildings, roads, trees, all spread out like a rainbow carpet and coming towards me faster and faster, getting bigger by the second.

Back down on the ground, everything I've been through seems to leave my soul. I can't remember anything. Later that evening, it all comes flooding back to me. Wonderful. So glad when the DVD and photos come back. One of my goals achieved!

A decade later and my life had moved on in so many different ways, but I wanted to prove to myself and others I still had the balls and confidence to chuck myself out of a plane AGAIN!

Didn't just do this once, nor twice, but three times. Still asking why. Secretly, I know, because it is me – I can do anything I want to.

I'm Free

High above the clouds
And back down to Earth
Freedom, empowerment, in control
Back down with a bump
I was still on cloud nine though!

Ten years on - broken bones
With a hubby and a Mummy of two
But still no fear
I wanted to prove I still had it in me

Flying high above the clouds
The adrenaline rush came flooding back
And I was set free
Once again from this spastic body

Firmly back on the ground
I was overjoyed to be amongst the clouds
For a few minutes
But I needed to find my way back
To the booking office

And book a third jump
Barmy, mad, crazy, stupid
Or brave, courageous and fearless
Whatever the word
That's me!

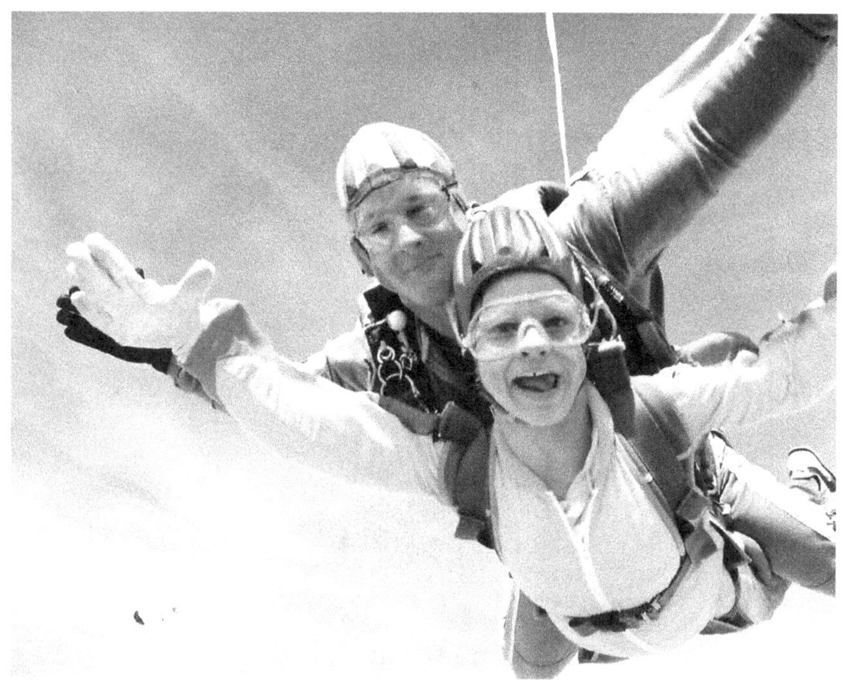

My first jump

My Life

It's my life
Nobody else's
But mine
Choices
Fuck ups
High and lows
Hopes and dreams
Sadness and disappointment
Everyone has their say
In my life
But why?
I don't have a say
In their life
Able mind
My life
No one else's
Add one simple word
Spastic
And it's everyone's life
Everyone seems to think
They should be part of it

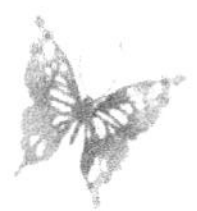

'You do know what's wrong with your daughter, don't you?'

Born on October 31st, 1973, just before midnight, I'm a typical Scorpio. Friends call me fiery, passionate, unforgiving sometimes. I wear my heart on my sleeve. Scorpios are like that. Probably give my heart to anyone who needs it, but upset or use me only once! I don't give half, I give full … but can get hurt that way. I don't know how to hold back.

Date and the time of my birth are the easy bit. Mum and Dad have told me what happened that day, but those early years are like an album with lots of photos missing. Did they tell me everything? What would the missing photographs show? This is what I do know. Parents Simon and Trish were soldiers in the British Army, stationed in Germany and already had Logan, my three-year-old sister. Mum said it was a straightforward pregnancy with no problems. I imagine she was looking forward to a sister or brother for Logan. So far, so perfect. An ordinary, 'normal' family.

My parents were in their late 20s when I came along. What happened on the night of my birth turned us from a typical young family into something very different. That night had a huge impact on our family and our friends forever and, of course, on me.

Dad took Mum off to the military hospital when she went into labour. Pictures I've seen of the place look pretty grim. She wasn't expecting any problems. Being a second child, I imagine she thought it would be a piece of cake.

First problem was that no-one believed Mum was in labour. Instead, they put it down to a urine infection. She was made to march up and down the corridor. I don't know why. Neither did she. They kept her in and sent Dad home. Next thing he heard was a phone call at midnight asking him to come to the hospital urgently as his wife was critically ill and new baby was in an incubator.

Mum had been in labour for 36 hours and, when I eventually pushed my way into the world, I was blue. Looking at the medical records, I just want to scream at someone and say: 'Why didn't you do something to help my Mum? Why didn't you know immediately something was wrong with me?' Believe it or not, they didn't think anything was.

Mum and Dad took me home, where Mum was like a single parent. Dad was posted here, there and everywhere and she just got on with it. She knew something wasn't right because Logan was a 'normal' baby, but just got on as best she could. She didn't know what to do which, in a weird way, was a positive. Not having a 'label' for me, she had me potty-trained and sitting up, stuff like that.

She went back and forth to hospital in Germany but was just fobbed off. People weren't listening. For almost the first three years of my life in Germany, Mum coped as best she could. She plugged away at the authorities and finally got a transfer back to the UK to take me to specialists and find out what was wrong. She took me to Charing Cross Hospital because I had a dislocated hip – a common thing in children with cerebral palsy. But she didn't think anything of it because my sister had had one.

I was apparently sitting on the floor, struggling to put some stick-a-bricks together, when the paediatrician said: "You do know what's wrong with your daughter, don't you?"

So, now, we knew. I was three and we finally had a diagnosis of cerebral palsy. Except he didn't say cerebral palsy, he said spastic. That's what we were called in those days. Nobody thought anything of it. Mum didn't know about CP but definitely knew what a spastic was. She was instantly aware of what she was taking on. It was a huge relief that someone finally acknowledged what she had been saying was true. 'Your daughter is a spastic!' the doctor said, but Mum knew I had capabilities and wasn't stupid. In contrast, when my parents told my extended family, there was a sharp intake of breath, a really negative reaction. 'She's disabled!' They wanted to wrap me in cotton wool.

Mum hates injustice and my birth was a great injustice. Someone did something wrong, but nothing was admitted. Mum fought battle after battle. I think I inherited her determination. When I was about four and attending a special needs school in London, they wanted to take me with a group of kids on a residential stay to Hayling Island. I wanted to go, too, but Mum panicked. Teachers persuaded her I'd be fine and I just blossomed. Awful show off, you see!

Sister

I can, I will and I do
I might be different to you but I can still make it through
Cerebral palsy makes it more challenging and rewarding
I don't know any different
I will always be strong and hold my head up high
I'm just like you, I'm able
It might be different to you, but I will always achieve my goals

Exercise and physio improved my physical abilities a lot between the ages of 5 and 10 and I was able to walk with sticks and a walking frame. It was tiring and not very practical if we wanted to go any distance. One of my first really strong memories as a child was being so excited because I was getting my first wheelchair. How sad is that when I was aged just five? Sounds strange, but it meant freedom and independence.

Until then, I was either struggling with my sticks or frame or in a buggy – a too-big child in a buggy. Dead giveaway, isn't it? I see them now when I go into town --kids too big and too old for a buggy - and you just know they're not quite right.
My new wheelchair was bright orange and green. We went on holiday to Torquay where Dad's family lived and he got a parking ticket. We put it on my wheelchair. I was so proud of that wheelchair. I covered it in Mickey Mouse stickers. I also had a walking frame and felt just like my sister.

Getting my First Wheels

I'm going to be a proper little girl,
I'm going to be able,
I'm going to be free,
I'm going to join in,
I'm going to be big and strong,
I'm going to sit up tall and be counted as me,
I'm not an oversized baby in a buggy,
I'm Kerry and I just happen to have cerebral palsy,
My bright orange chair will take me where I need.

I could walk, felt like a proper little girl, normal. While I was thrilled to bits with my wheelchair, it was completely different for my parents. I think it was a sad time for Mum and Dad because the wheelchair meant my disability was 'out there'. The move from buggy to wheelchair was powerful for me, but a lot for them to cope with after having an able-bodied child first.

My parents tried to sue the army over my birth when I was six but didn't get anywhere. Looking back, I had a happy childhood with a family who cared about me ... and I had my freedom chair. Probably wasn't until I was about eight that I first felt 'disabled' or not quite as 'able'.

Logan was out playing with her friends and Mum was in the kitchen. I crawled into the room to see her and sat on my hands. "Why can't I go out with Logan? Why? Why? Why?' As I screamed and cried, Mum said I "shouldn't worry about what I couldn't do but be grateful she was there to care for me because otherwise I wouldn't be able to do anything". She carried on washing up with tears running down her face as I pleaded, "Please don't tell Daddy." I was worried he'd be angry I'd upset her. That's when I knew I would never be like my sister.

My parents never told me back then what was actually wrong with me. They never said: "You've got cerebral palsy and this is what it means." I resent that. I would rather have known. When I was about 10, I wanted to be a hairdresser! Imagine the kind of haircut you'd get with me suddenly having a spasm?! If you came out alive, that is! Spastics and scissors don't really mix!

Of course, they said I couldn't do that, but never told me why. These days we talk about everything, but it was different back then. I knew I was different and not 'normal' because I went to a special school, where most of the kids were in wheelchairs and a special bus picked me up, whilst my sister went to the local school and had lots of friends from the nearby streets. I didn't have any nearby friends because they were bussed to my school from all over the place. I had to rely on my sister and her friends. She hated that, her friends resented me, and I hated it too.

Logan struggled because of my disability. Because of it, however unwanted, I had extra attention. People worried about me and spent more time and effort on my care. We both found the situation very difficult. If only I could have told my sister I wanted to be like her. We didn't get on.

What It's Like to Be Me

I didn't want to be like this,
I didn't choose it but I've got this
I'm able, strong and determined,
It's what's inside that counts,
Having CP has made me who I am
I'm strong, determined, fiery, bubbly
Nothing beats me,
I find a way
It might be different but it's my way
It's my life and it's my CP
It comes with me; I don't go with it!

I joined the local weekly Red Cross group that met in the town centre. It was brilliant. I fitted in straightaway; everybody accepted me for who I was. I felt I belonged and was happy and content. Like the other kids, I worked towards badges and achieved my first aid badge. I was so proud.

I guess you're wondering how I managed to put someone in the recovery position?! So was I! They would probably have ended up worse off! But I could explain how to do it. On the day of the exam, it was decided I would ask someone I didn't know to carry out the physical part. This proved more difficult than first thought but I passed and went on to gain several more badges. I was beginning to outgrow the Red Cross group and wanted to look for alternative options within the community.

Having already been involved in Brownies at my special school, I attended a special needs Girl Guide camp which I loved. I was able to be myself joining in with all the activities and trying new ones. I volunteered as the main pot cleaner using a Brillo pad, managing to get messier than the pots to start with. I had so much fun cleaning those pots and myself!

During the camp holiday when we were able to join in with the cooking on the campfire, I took the lead role toasting the marshmallows. This was going brilliantly until I had a spasm when I saw the marsh mallows alight. To my horror, I placed the marshmallows on somebody's shoulder! That so happened to belong to a visitor wanting to know more about disability. She certainly learnt the hard way!

After the pack holiday, I really liked the idea of joining a local Girl Guides group. I was going to be the only disabled girl in the pack, but this made it more exciting. I knew I could do it having just left the Red Cross after gaining all my badges.

After doing some research, we decided I would join the local guides close to my home. The captain welcomed me with open arms and soon lots of girls were collecting me from my home and walking together to the meetings. It felt brilliant being accepted by the Guides. I worked hard towards my badges, just like the others, and achieved everything a Girl Guide should.

I found learning to sew very difficult, but I did it! No matter how big a challenge I set myself, I achieve my aims. Sewing was certainly different to the others. I enjoyed Guides for several months and looked forward to those few hours a week where I could show off the skills I was fast learning. It brought me a sense of freedom and belonging.

However, due to ill health, the captain could no longer manage and the new captain took an instant dislike to me. She took Dad aside and told him I was no longer fitting in with the group and couldn't sew! She said the girls would eventually reject me and I had to leave. Dad, as always, took it in his stride and, unknown to me, went home and told Mum. She collected me from that meeting and had a few choice words to say to the captain!

Mum had to explain to me why I was no longer able to be a Girl Guide. I was heartbroken and devastated. I could sew and join in and loved being with the girls. I felt normal. It must have been the hardest thing for Mum and I couldn't comprehend it as I lived for those meetings. Suddenly I wasn't able to go.

This was another major injustice for Mum and for me. She wasn't going to let it lie and contacted the local paper and the

Guiding Association to air her views. A few days later, my headteacher told me I couldn't go on a school trip as reporters, from not only the local paper but the BBC, were coming to interview me!

The BBC had me sewing during the interview and it was aired on the News at One. Little did I know that this wouldn't be the last time that I'd be on the BBC! After the publicity, I was invited to join another Girl Guide group in my town. It was brilliant but never the same as it was located in the town centre and was too far for the girls to walk with me. That was the first – but definitely not the last – time I experienced discrimination because I was disabled.

For all that spasms have dominated my life, the thing I really hate is I have deafness in both ears. This obviously affects my speech and impacts on the way other people react to me. My parents took me for a hearing test when I was 10 and I was given a hearing aid, which I promptly threw down the toilet. It was the last thing I wanted. I felt – rightly or wrongly – that with a hearing aid and unclear speech, people would think I was stupid. I also felt that a hearing aid picked up too much background noise.

I am great at lip reading now and I get by. But if you asked me what my greatest disabilities are, I would probably say my deafness and people's attitudes.

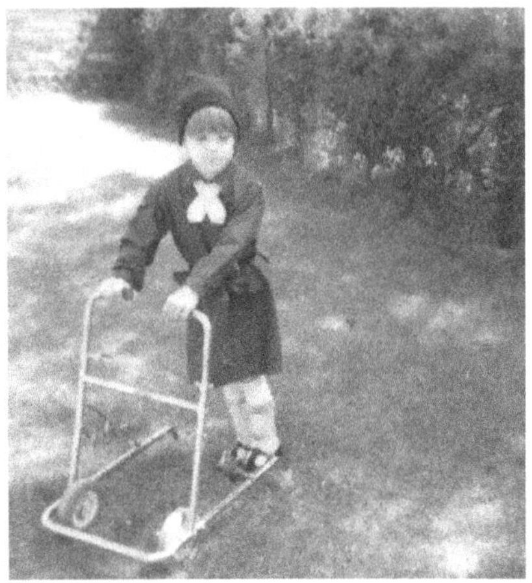

Age 6 in my Brownie uniform

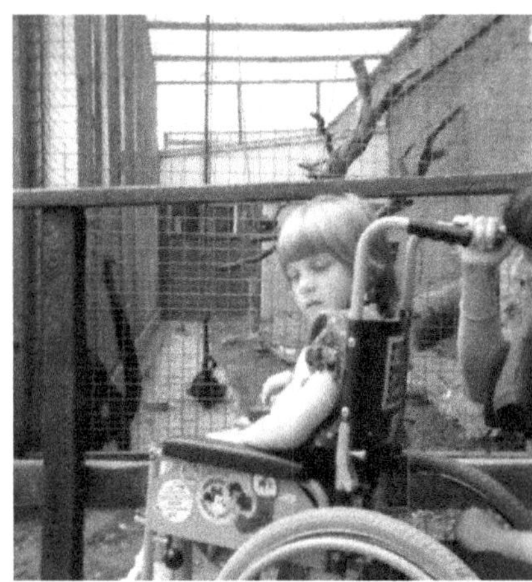

Age 6 in my amazing wheelchair

Health

Cerebral Palsy first on the list!
Not bad, can't hear, can't walk
Can't move normally
Loads of spasms
Stiff
Weak
Uncoordinated
Deaf as a post
Apart from that, normal!
I'm a woman
Mood swings
Periods
Body change
Apart from that, normal!

Or am I?

Living With CP

I always knew I was different but didn't know how different until I was about six or seven.

I started to wonder why I couldn't do things like everyone else. Yes, I had two arms, two legs, a head etc and that made me a person. Yet my body seemed to work in a different way. It was almost like a computer that wasn't programmed properly. My brain wasn't wired up to my body parts. God only knows what this was called – no one would tell me. I had to learn the hard way how my body moved and operated. It was like I was a teacher and pupil! I suppose, in a way, it helped me not knowing much as I was able to push my body to the limits.

My cerebral palsy is kind of fun in a strange way as I tend to move into odd and peculiar positions and wonder how the hell I got there! Having spasms - a contraction of the muscles that tense up and is extremely painful, lasting from minutes to hours - I have had to learn several techniques of how to deal with them and know my own body and its capabilities.

Over the years, I've tried some weird and wonderful ways of getting out of spasm. I've tried shaking my limbs and someone physically sitting on top of me – both methods work really well, but I'm not advising anyone to do it! It's just what works best for you – you are the expert on your own body.

Throughout the years, I've found sudden noise makes me jump if I'm not expecting it. I've learnt ways to adapt to this, such as blocking out all the background noise. Listening to music certainly helps a great deal and alleviates all the erratic movements.

Life is certainly a challenge with CP but, to be fair, I don't know any different. I've lived with my body for the past 40 odd years. Yes, it is a challenge, and some days are better than others. It's particularly different in extreme weather conditions and when temperatures suddenly change from hot to cold or vice versa.

At the end of the day you learn to live with what you've got. I've grown up in the same body I was born in and I'll die with that body. So, you could say I'm the expert on me. I'm not sure how my CP will affect me later in life and how my spasms and movements will change but I'm determined to carry on without relying too heavily on medication.

I do use Botox – in my face, of course! – every six months in my right side to help with the pain and discomfort. This allows me to live and maintain an independent life. I use an electric wheelchair full time as I have knackered my body over the years living an able-bodied life in a spastic body.

But I wouldn't change a thing. I wouldn't have had the same opportunities if I hadn't pushed my body to the extreme. I often get asked by kids what it's like to have CP. I find that quite a challenging and difficult question to answer as I don't know what it's like not to have CP. I often answer: 'What's it like to be able-bodied?'

Everyone who has CP is unique and different in every way – no two people are the same. It depends on the individual and how they cope with the challenges of having CP. I'm very fortunate as I'm able to communicate and of high intelligence. One thing's for sure, having CP has made me a much stronger person. You need to have a wicked sense of humour and make every challenge possible. It's not often I get down and mope about but, if I do, I always remember someone is worse off than myself. I pick myself up and carry on to my next challenge.

I've always been bloody strong minded and determined to succeed in everything I do – and that goes for my physical needs. At the end of the day, I don't know what it's like to be you. I know what it's like to be me. If it takes me two hours to get dressed, then that's how long it takes. At least I've accomplished it on my own and that's my dignity, self-worth and confidence.

I always hold to the motto that 'I can do it' and this has been embedded with me throughout the years.

School Years

Those were the good old days
School years
Best days of your life
Or were they?
Hospital school
Fixing the problem
Making it right for society
We are kids after all
We need to have fun
We need to learn
We need to play
We need to laugh
We need friends
We need school
We need education!

Where do I start? I'm sitting here reminiscing about my school days, finding it very difficult as it was many years ago! I have mixed emotions about school as my school years began three years after being diagnosed with cerebral palsy and lasted to the grand age of 16!

During such a huge chunk of my life, I had some amazing experiences. Some happy, some sad, some challenging, some thought-provoking. I went through a lot of heartache, frustration and disappointment, as well as happy, exciting, soul-searching times. I met some amazing and incredible people during the 11 years I spent at school.

I always remember my first school, if you can call it a school! My parents chose it as it catered for children with cerebral palsy and other disabilities. I needed a lot of input physically in the form of speech and physiotherapy after my diagnosis, and John Greenwood Shipman School seemed to be the answer.

Situated in the heart of Northamptonshire, it was an old Victorian house surrounded by spectacular gardens. It's what I would describe as a 'hospital school', mainly concentrating on the physical needs of a child as opposed to academic ability. It was very regimented with a lot of emphasis being placed on all the therapies, rather than reading, writing and arithmetic.

Special schools were few and far between. You may only have found one in a whole county. Therefore, children were often shipped in by school transport from their homes, which could be up to 20 miles away. This was the case for me, so my school day started at 7:45am and finished at 4:45pm. I didn't get to school until 9:30am! I had a wonderful driver who picked four of us up in a car every morning and brought us back home in the evening. We called him Uncle Tom. He became part of the family and made the journey go really quickly, listening to Jungle Book all the way. I really looked forward to the mornings and, after five years, knew the words of Jungle Book off by heart!

When we arrived at school, our regime started with physiotherapy, then a walk up the corridor using my rollator. About seven metres on, without being asked, I was led to a toilet. It was presumed I needed to go. It took about 15 minutes to complete the task. I eventually arrived at my classroom just in time for lunch! Afterwards, I was led into the bathroom for another wee. I didn't realise cerebral palsy gave you a weak bladder! Nine times out of 10 I didn't even need to go! I was led back into the classroom to watch tele before uncle Tom came to pick us up.

That's how my days went for several years. Luckily, my teacher Miss Mills came to my rescue. This was her first teaching post and she saw potential in me. In the little time she had with me in the classroom, she encouraged me to learn to read and write. I gained confidence and started to believe in myself and my abilities. I really enjoyed being encouraged and stretched to achieve my academic ability.

Then John Greenwood Shipman School was closed and reopened as an old age pensioner residential home. I've already put my name down for a place when I'm older! I was sent to another special school, this time closer to home – only 10 miles away! Again, I used school transport including pick-ups and drop offs, still at ridiculous times. But, for me, Kingsley was a proper school. It followed the National Curriculum, had school assemblies, and we did PE, cooking and science. Wow! I was 10 years old and excited to go to school. I still concentrated on my therapies and was made to walk to my lessons, but I felt like a real schoolgirl and that was important to me.

To Leah

Loveable

Educator

Achiever

Happiness

From the first moment you stepped into the room
I knew we just clicked
You need me I need you
You are my inspiration
You are my guide
You are my belief
I can count on you
No matter what

You know what to do
You know what to say
You know how to be strong when I'm low

You know how to drive me through when storms are blue
I love you, Leah!

I'll always remember my first day at Kingsley. I felt scared and lost. There were only 100 pupils in the school ranging from 3 to 16 years old, but this was a big leap from John Greenwood, as they had 30 pupils in total! Kingsley catered for a whole range of disabilities, including cerebral palsy, spina bifida, epilepsy, and other multiple health conditions. My teacher asked me which was my left and right. I felt so embarrassed as no one had taught me. I genuinely thought that, if you turned around, your left became your right and right became your left!

I enjoyed school, and in the first few years picked up ways teachers taught their pupils. I discovered really quickly that some praised effort as opposed to quality. I decided to put this theory to the test. I produced a really crap piece of work - I knew it wasn't my best - and presented it to the teacher, who then praised me for the work! I felt so disappointed, let down and confused, it was untrue. Had I been able-bodied, I would have been made to do the work again but, because the teacher had seen the physical effort as opposed to anything else, I was praised for it. My ability certainly wasn't stretched, and I became lazy and thought to myself, 'Why am I bothering?' as no one was taking me seriously.

When I was 11, everything just seemed to kick off. It was an emotional and challenging time, entering into my teenage years, especially knowing that some teachers and support staff were not seeing past my disability and seeing me for me. However, much to my delight, the head teacher introduced 2 amazing and supportive teachers to her team. First being Kev Thompson, a new Drama teacher. Second, Leah Stirrat, a new English and Humanities teacher- both with their own individual qualities and expertise.

Kevan, or then known as Mr Thompson to me, was a breath of fresh air and was up for any challenge which was presented to him. He got everyone involved with school productions and going on walking and camping expeditions. Nothing seems to faze him. He saw beyond our disabilities and captured our capabilities. He was all-singing, all-dancing, all the way! Just what we all needed to rise above our physical barriers and see our full potential.

Another amazing teacher was Leah. She had little or no experience of working with youngsters with disabilities and therefore no preconceived ideas of what we could achieve academically. Leah instantly saw beyond our disabilities and realised our abilities. I took a real shine to this new teacher and built up a rapport with her.

I decided to test the boundaries and put her to the test. Leah set us a challenge and I handed in a really crap piece of work and waited for her response. To my shock, amazement, astonishment and excitement, the response I'd waited to hear finally came back! She said to me: "I think you did this in front of the TV! And if you want to achieve in the real world you need to show what you can do … They don't have special stickers saying 'done by a girl with CP, she needs extra marks…'" I was so taken aback and overjoyed with her response that a great bond formed between us.

We worked together to achieve anything we wanted because she believed in me and I believed in her. I worked my butt off to prove to myself and others I was just as able as any other young person who wanted the same things in life. We set our goals high and worked hard towards my GCSEs. It was incredible, especially when you think I started the school five years earlier not knowing my left from my right. I really did feel I was part of the able-bodied world and achieving my goals. I was tested, challenged and stretched academically, emotionally and physically. I knew, with the help and support of this very special lady, I could do anything. She filled me with confidence, self-esteem and self-belief, and made me feel counted. I wasn't just a disabled teenager. I was Kerry.

I was becoming independent at home and venturing into town on my own. It soon became apparent I couldn't access the local shopping centre without someone having to push the fire doors open for me. I was extremely disappointed. It didn't make sense that the shopping centre had ramps inside but no electric doors! I took matters into my own hands. I wrote a letter to the manager of the centre explaining my situation and disappointment, highlighting the fact that it wasn't just disabled people but old people and mothers with pushchairs and people in general who had difficulty gaining access. However, much to my horror and disappointment, I received a letter from the manager within a day to say they had no plans to install electric doors.

I felt let down and angry he wasn't taking the situation seriously. So, I tried again. The next day I designed a petition sheet. For the next four Saturdays, I sat outside the shopping centre with a little coffee table collecting signatures for my campaign. I managed to obtain 1435 signatures and, on the last Saturday, handed in my petition to the manager. Two days later I received a letter asking my parents and I to attend a meeting with the manager to discuss the matter.

During the first part of the meeting, he directed his questions towards my parents. I was angry and upset, as he obviously thought they had put me up to this. I made it perfectly clear that it was my project, my idea, my independence at stake. After he realised the campaign was solely my idea, his attitude changed and he focused the conversation on me instead of my parents. Again, I had changed and challenged people's attitudes around disability. I was overjoyed to find that electric doors were installed at the shopping centre six weeks later.

Another fun and exciting opportunity I was involved with was when I was 14 and working alongside teenage boys from a mainstream school on a garden project. We wanted to create a wheelchair accessible garden. We had the ideas but not the physical skills or abilities to do it. The boys had the physical ability, so we worked together to achieve our goal. Again, this broke down barriers and changed and challenged attitudes towards disability. It was an incredible and unique friendship that lasted for years.

This project also led me to receive a grant from the Prince's Trust to fund the project. I was nominated for Best of British Youth for my efforts and contribution and couldn't believe it when I came fourth out of 500 people. I went to the Savoy Hotel in London and met celebrities such as Frank Bough, Moira Gray and Kid Jensen. I also had the opportunity to do a live interview on Sky Television that night. It was an incredible experience, and I had the most wonderful opportunity to represent the school as well as learning about myself.

I was beginning to look to the future and what I wanted to do when I left school two years later. Opportunities for disabled teenagers were very limited and often decided by professionals such as teachers and social workers. Being strong minded and determined, I conducted my own research and explored opportunities outside the county. I really thought I hadn't had the same opportunities as my able-bodied sister during her teenage years, due to my cerebral palsy and having to rely on others for my care.

I wanted to gain further GCSEs and greater freedom and independence. It became apparent that the three other colleges in the county weren't suitable for my requirements. One was a residential placement but seemed like John Greenwood Shipman - lovely big house, beautiful gardens, but was this really suitable for a teenager? I think not! I wanted pubs, shops and able-bodied people around me. Was that too much to ask for?

I also looked into day college placement, but that was a dumping ground. All the disabled students were put together in a special unit, doing meaningless tasks. It was an insult to our ability and intelligence. I had already done a term of one afternoon a week and they made me transfer buttons from one box to another. This, too, was a meaningless task, especially as I had cerebral palsy and my hand coordination was shit, but I was determined to complete it. I completed one such task way before the allocated time, so they made me put all the buttons back in the same box! I couldn't see myself surviving a day, let alone two years of this crap. I deserved so much more. I was studying for my

GCSEs and there was no way I was going to be patronised and go backwards.

Looking at out-of-county provision, I came across three residential colleges. We decided to look at all of them. Two colleges were located in fantastic grounds, surrounded by several acres of land but where were the pubs, shops, clubs or cinemas? Would you expect an able-bodied teenager to want to go to a college like this? So why expect a disabled teenager to go there?

I found a brilliant college situated in the heart of Coventry. Hereward College was the answer to all my dreams and aspirations. The location was a fantastic bus route away from the town centre, two minutes from the local pub and five minutes from the shops. To top it all, Hereward College was adjacent to Tower Hill mainstream College, so students had the best of both worlds.

Hereward provided 24-hour care and support provision in independent rooms and flats, as well as offering students the chance to further their academic studies. Sounded absolutely fantastic. I made up my mind Hereward was the place I wanted to be. I just had to convince the local authority this would be cost effective and select the best academic programme for my needs. I was already following a plan at school aiming to achieve three GCSEs, which was bloody marvellous considering where I started my academic studies and mainly due to sheer determination and the influence of Leah.

It is really unusual for pupils to attend their own 14+ reviews but I was determined to be present. I just thought, if professionals were going to talk about me and my future, it was only right I was there to put my case forward! After a lengthy meeting and some correspondence, it was decided I would go for a trial at Hereward College to see how I got on. This included an overnight assessment of my needs and an academic interview.

I was really excited to be offered the chance to excel myself and quickly got to work choosing my further GCSE subjects. This was the time when the BT advert was on the tele where Maureen Lipman rings her grandson about his GCSE results and the only one he got was in sociology. "You've got an ology, you can be a doctor!" It sounded fantastic and the fact

I couldn't say 'sociology' made me more determined to study the subject! My second choice was law, mainly because I thought it was above me and would be really interesting. Also it seemed to work well with sociology. My third choice, welfare in society, was taught at Tile Hill as opposed to Hereward. I wanted the chance to mix with able-bodied students and to become a social worker.

My choices made, all I had to do was sit back and wait for a decision. It seemed like the longest time in my life, as I had set my heart on going to Hereward, but knew I had to get my head down to achieve my three GCSEs and prove to myself and others Hereward was the right placement for me. The decision finally came through and I would be able to have out-of- county provision at Hereward College. I was ecstatic, overjoyed, couldn't believe my luck. I was determined to make the most of every opportunity my new challenge threw at me. I felt lost, apprehensive, scared and confused as well as excited to be a normal teenager.

I was leaving home to join the big wide world!

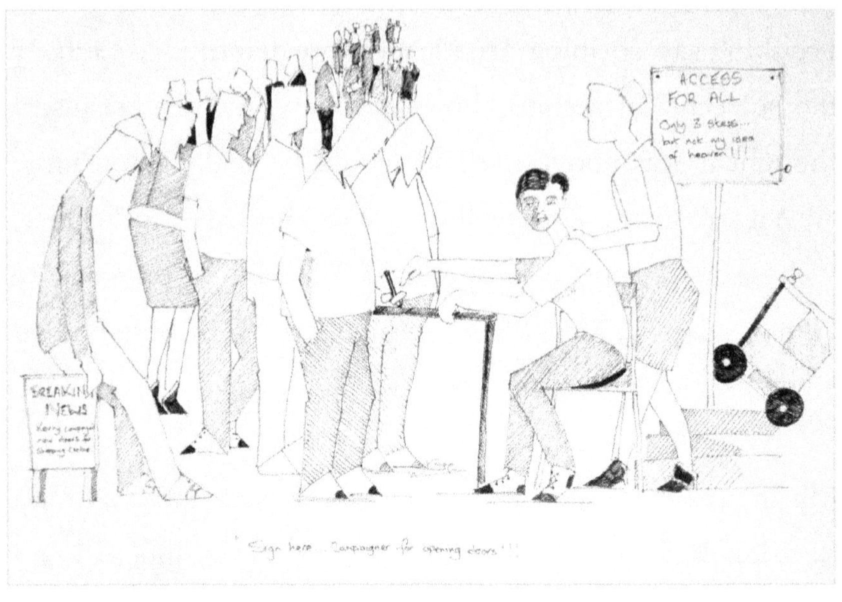
ACCESS
FOR ALL
Only 3 steps...
but not my idea
of heaven!!!
BREAKIN
NEWS
"Sign here... Campaigner for opening doors!!!

Holidays

Holiday, residentials, time out
You decide!
For me it was a time of freedom
Experimenting independence
And discovering who Kerry is

It all comes with a price
Planning, organizing, developing
School holidays were the best
Away with friends Experimenting and having fun
It's got to be done
Disabled or not

Holidays, like everything else, are not always straightforward, especially when your name is Kerry!

As a child, we had many family holidays, both within the UK and abroad. We were lucky that our grandparents lived by the seaside, so we enjoyed happy times there. We also spent time with our grandparents at Butlins whilst my parents enjoyed going on holiday themselves. This enabled my sister and I to get up to all kinds of mischief without panicking or stressing out our parents. Bags of fun, adventure and chaos!
I remember such a holiday where we had been to the funfair and the weather was glorious. After dragging Nan and Grandad around all the rides it was time to head home, singing and laughing all the way, the five of us – my three cousins, my sister and I - full of beans. But we failed to notice a big black cloud behind us! The cloud followed us for about five minutes until it gave in and burst and we all got drowned. It was so much fun.

Then the sun reappeared and we all started to dry off - brilliant for my sister and cousins who were able to walk and dry themselves quicker but not so much for a wet girl in a wheelchair with spasms coming into play. However, we tried to make the best of our worst nightmare and continued singing and messing around until we got home. Nan made us a hot chocolate and a bath and I was soon out of spasm and tucked up in bed remembering the highlights of the day. Other childhood holidays included going abroad. One such memory was when I was six and we went to Portugal for a week. I remember always winning at bingo. Looking back I think it was a fix but I was overjoyed and kept on buying drinks at the bar with my winnings! I didn't feel disabled, I just felt like a big girl!

When I was 11, we went to Benidorm on our first all-inclusive family holiday. After checking the accommodation, it was decided to go ahead with the holiday. To our dismay, when we turned up at the hotel, it was located on a massive hill! It was brilliant going down, but someone always had to push me back up. On the third day my sister tried the all-inclusive cocktails and ended up very paralytic, falling over and twisting her ankle. She was bandaged up at hospital and had to rely on a wheelchair to get around. We got some stares on that holiday with two youngsters in wheelchairs! We continued to see the funny side of it and made the most of the holiday. We made the best of sight-seeing, sunbathing and generally enjoying our family holiday together.

Another cherished memory was a family holiday to Africa. Teachers and friends had dared me to go on a camel. Like I say when Kerry sets her mind, Kerry always achieves! I managed to get on the bloody camel, admittedly not for long. The camel took some steps with me on his back so to me I rode a camel… admittedly it was only 6! Oh my! Getting on… bloody nightmare! My dad was pushing, my mum was pulling, my cousin was laughing… and I was farting and spasming! But between us we managed to do it and I rode that bloody camel! Another box ticked.

During my childhood years I ventured out on my own with different groups and school residentials. I was involved with an organization called PHAB (Physically Handicapped Able-Bodied- it was the 1980s after all). But what are words? I think people hide behind labels and don't concentrate on the important stuff in life. I was born and will die a spastic, nothing will change that, so why get bogged down with political correctness?

Anyway, where was I? Oh yeah, I was on a PHAB holiday

and it was fab! Away from my family and no one knowing my capabilities, not even myself. A week of freedom, discovery, excitement and no sleep! We were paired with an able-bodied young person to achieve challenges and activities together. As always, I was the first disabled youngster to go rock climbing and abseiling. I was nervous as hell but determined not to let this stop me. I went potholing and canoeing and excelled myself gaining in confidence and self- esteem. Such experiences lasted for years. The instructor was pushing and I was holding on for dear life, trying hard not to fart in his face! At the same time laughing hysterically.

My first ever school residential was when I was just four and a half years old. My parents were really nervous at allowing me to go at such an early age but I am so grateful that they did as this gave me the confidence, determination and self-esteem that has enabled me to achieve my goals. These trips became an annual event in the school calendar. Such trips ranged from overnight stays at a local youth hostel to a whole week camping and a stay on a narrow boat. These weeks were absolutely fantastic, being away from home and experiencing new and exciting challenges. We were able to test the boundaries and be as independent as we possibly could without being judged by family members, and also rising to the challenge our teachers set us knowing that they knew only too well what we were capable of. Sometimes you can kid your parents but you can't kid your teachers! Furthermore, I was with friends I didn't usually see outside of school. We had a ball, trying new activities, pushing our disabled bodies to the limit, which I loved. Who knows what can be achieved until you have conquered your goals and fears? My school trips were the best times. We forgot about our disabilities and concentrated on our abilities. We always found a way around our challenge and for me it was a sense of achievement, a sense of belonging, a sense of freedom and empowerment.

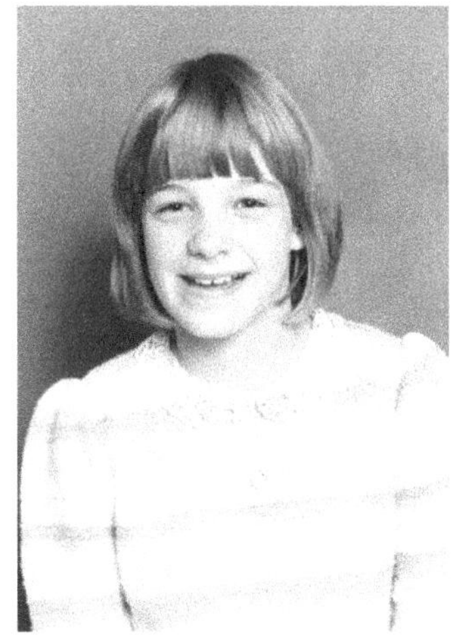
Me age 6

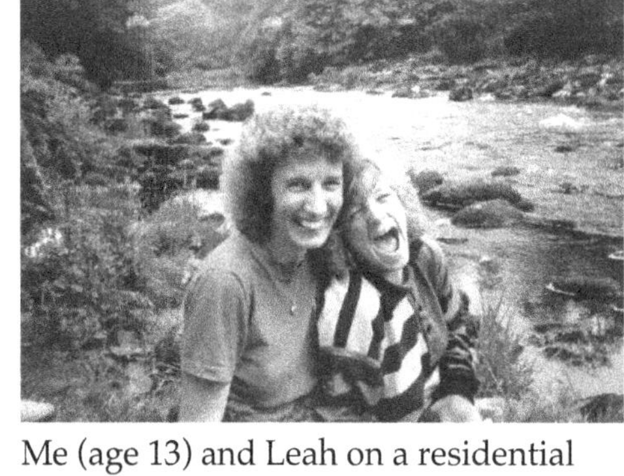
Me (age 13) and Leah on a residential

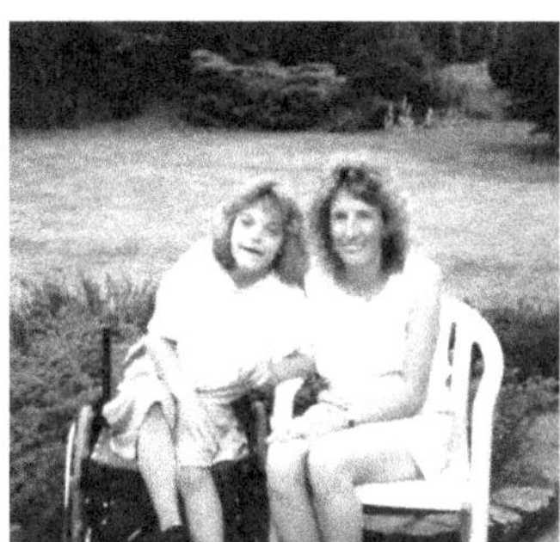
Me and Leah, age 14

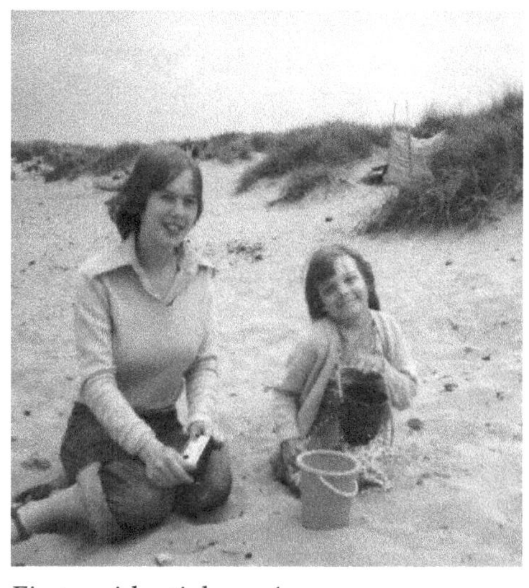
First residential age 4

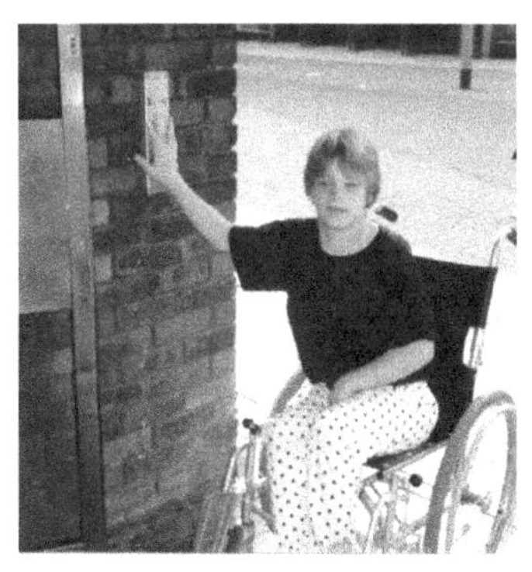
Electric doors!

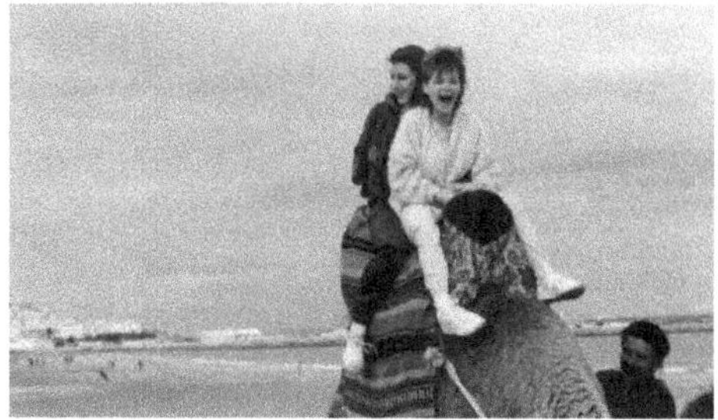
Camel Riding

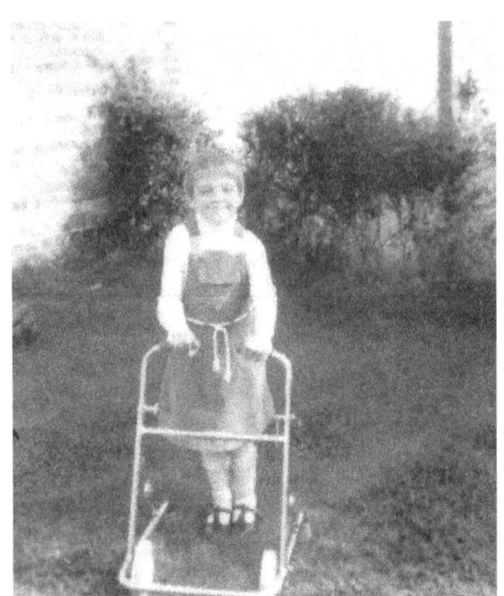

Me and my rollator, age 7

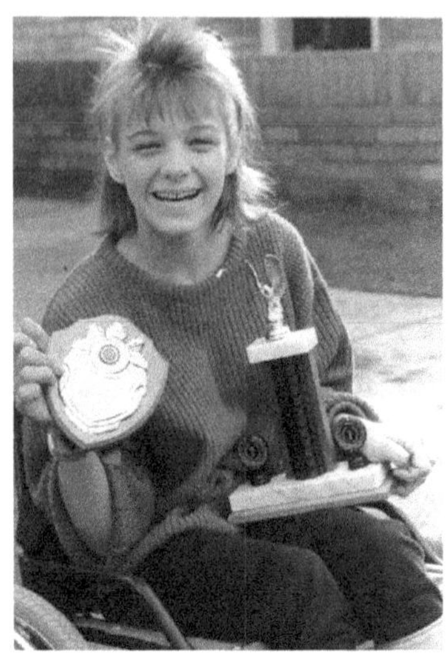

Archery awards, aged 15

Teenage Years

I'm confused
I feel trapped, lonely, frustrated
I don't know which way to turn
And when I do
I don't know who to ask or what to say
Am I still me?
Am I someone else?
Changes in my body Changes in my mind
Who can help me?
No one's telling me which way to go
I'm still a spastic
Will I be in this body for life?
I need to know
I need to understand
It's just part of life, isn't it?
I will get there I always do

Teenage years are often the most complex and challenging time of a young person's life with many questions unanswered and this is no exception for a disabled teenager. In fact, it could be said that this is a double whammy as it is certainly a challenging and soul-searching time. It may be a period where you have to come to terms with body change as well as realising the impact of being different. Time to brave a difficult period of my life and share my experience of teenage years. Self-discovery, realisation, loneliness and confusion.

My body was developing into a woman and I wanted to be as physically independent as possible, whilst still having to rely heavily on my parents. I couldn't just jump in the bath for as long as I wanted when my body was crying out for help in spasm. I didn't understand then what a spasm was and how it affected me. I thought everyone had spasms.

I was becoming too heavy for Mum to lift me in and out of the bath, so Dad had to do it. I resorted to wearing my swimsuit to protect my dignity, as well as his. My bath routine usually took two to three hours to complete.

Therefore baths were restricted to three a week. Deep down I knew the reason why, but it didn't stop me feeling angry and frustrated. My family tried their best and I suppose it was frustrating for them too. I felt such a burden during those years and I suppose they felt the same. I couldn't just walk out of the door, be with my friends and join in with other teenagers. I had to stay at home, look forward to having baths and deal with my physical care needs.

It was really frustrating. Why me? I didn't ask for this, didn't want anyone helping me with bathing and toileting. My sister didn't have this, so why should I have to cope with it? I felt like I couldn't be a proper teenager. I couldn't join in with friends who lived miles away outside school hours and didn't really have friends at home as I was the only disabled child in the community. I just wanted to be normal, or was I?

I didn't fully understand what cerebral palsy meant and how it affected me. I honestly thought I'd wake up one day and be able to walk, talk normally and join in. No one had the nerve to sit me down and tell me that this was my life - born with CP, you die with CP!

My early ambition was to be a hairdresser. God, could you imagine the hairstyles? They would definitely have been unique! I just wanted to know what cerebral palsy was and how I was going to learn to survive with it. I was crying out for someone to tell me and help me along the way. My body was changing and my cerebral palsy was being dragged along with it.

Cerebral Palsy is as individual as the person, no two people are the same. There are three main types of Cerebral Palsy – athetoid, spastic and ataxic. All three can have different degrees of severity. One person could possess all three types but one could be very mild and the others very major. It's an individual disability and you never know what anyone can achieve. Cerebral Palsy also has associated disabilities such as epilepsy, a learning disability and/or a hearing impairment. I have the latter and tend to use this to my own advantage - selective deafness, I think it's called!

I have a middle tone range of deafness, which mainly affects my literacy. I was made to wear my hearing aid in one ear for years. Ten years later, they decided to swap ears, as they couldn't decide if it was helping me. I was fuming as they hadn't asked me any questions before swapping the hearing aid. When they did so, I told them my name, address and age and they said: "There you go, you can hear better." I was so upset that was the last time I wore my hearing aid. Even 30 years later, I still manage to survive without it. I find it a bit annoying and frustrating, but always try to face people and use lip reading to help. Wherever there's a way, Kerry will find it!

No one explained to me what periods were before mine started at the vulnerable age of 11. I thought I'd got a tummy upset, gone into spasm and hadn't wiped myself properly. But, to my horror, the 'brown mess' kept on coming. I didn't know what to do. I waited until my next bath, then it was all out in the open that I'd started my periods.

My parents made me feel humiliated and embarrassed. They wanted to tell the world, going to the shop to equip me with everything I'd need. I wanted to shut myself away and cry. I'm sure most teenagers feel the same. I had no one to turn to. I thought of how I would manage going to the toilet on my own and keep this a secret. I managed quite well, considering the spasms and CP. I wore extra pants to stop leakage as double protection but hated wearing sanitary towels, which were bulky, annoying and uncomfortable. I wanted to be a normal teenage girl and use Tampax like my sister, but didn't know where to get the help and information I needed.

Where do teenage girls read up on such things as relationships and periods? Magazines are usually an answer but they were on the top shelves in my local newsagents and I felt embarrassed to ask someone to bring them down. Eventually I built up the courage to ask our school nurse to help and, after a long chat, I decided to try lil-lets. This created two problems - getting the things undone and making sure I didn't go into spasm and put them in the wrong place! I was so determined to conquer my challenge and show everybody I was just like a normal teenager that lil-lets became a normal monthly routine!

My first bra was another major highlight in my family's diary. But, for me, it was just another obstacle to my independence and a challenge to work around. I learnt to adapt well to my body change and having periods as well as surviving these challenging years.

One of the most challenging and complex issues of being a teenager attending a special school was losing my school friends. This seemed to be an integral part of special school life. Altogether I lost 11 school friends who died in my teenage years. It almost became the norm. But it certainly made me stronger and realise that death is just part of life. After one special person passed away, I became great friends with my next door neighbour's family and through them I met Steve.

Steve was in his early 20s when we met and dating my neighbour's daughter. Our friendship grew. He always saw past my disability and accepted me for me.

Together we've seen highs and lows, the darkest and happiest moments. After many years of friendship, Steve has become part of my family, always there in times of need, nothing too much trouble. Everyone needs a friend like Steve in their life.

I'm a very strong believer that the world is full of able-bodied people and you've got to get out there and be counted for you and be part of society. I was fortunate enough that my family refused to wrap me in cotton wool and allowed me to join in and be part of community life.

College Years

A time for experimenting
A time for testing
A time for discovery
A time for independence
A time for freedom
A time to be able
A time to be strong
A time to be free
A time to be me

Now for my college years and how they shaped me to become the person I am today. I was nervous, scared and excited like any 16-year-old about the next adventure. Especially as I'd chosen to leave home and start to enjoy my teenage years like my able-bodied counterparts. I just wanted to be normal and test the boundaries.

I chose Hereward College for two main reasons. Firstly, it was in the heart of the city of Coventry which would be good for my social life. It was also adjacent to a mainstream college, so I had the best of both worlds studying alongside able-bodied students and having my care and support needs looked after at Hereward.

Two of my GCSEs were based at Hereward, the other at Tile Hill. I was really excited about all of them but particularly welfare and society at Tile Hill. I longed to work alongside able-bodied teenagers and this was my chance to shine. I'm a very strong believer that the world is full of able-bodied people and, as a disabled person, feel I have to get out there and prove to myself and others that I'm just as able as my able-bodied counterpart. I feel that my abnormal body movements can and have a tendency to make people misjudge my intelligence. I personally feel that if I'm easy going about my CP and call myself a spastic it allows people to see past my disability and see the real Kerry, almost giving them permission to feel at ease in my presence. Whenever I'm confronted with negative/reluctant attitudes I always make the effort to challenge and change their "fear" towards difference. This is only my way of doing things but I strongly believe this is how I've broken down people's preconceived ideas about me.

I met amazing people, both able-bodied and disabled, in my first year at Tile Hill. I never thought I'd be sitting here writing about two of my closest friends I met there nearly 30 years ago! Janice and Fiona were and still are absolutely amazing and our friendships have gone from strength to strength. Both of them, like myself, were in their first year at college, vulnerable and naïve toward disability. I have to take my hat off to them as they both saw past my crazy but beautiful body and wanted to get to know the real Kerry. We formed a real special friendship. It's all so easy for able-bodied teenagers to shy away from disability if they have not been in direct contact with a disabled person, not knowing what level to aim the conversation at. This is often picked up by the older generation who may feel at ease with a disabled person's presence. Young people are our next generation and will say what they want to say and once it's all out in the open the preconceived barriers are inevitably broken down and great friendships are formed. Whenever we had a free period, we met at my flat or the students' union to enjoy each other's company.

We learnt together fast and formed a very strong and unique bond which has seen us all through the highs and lows of life, and we are still there to support each other now.

We had an amazing year together, learning and pushing the boundaries like any teenagers. For the first time in my life, I felt able and that people were taking me, for me, seeing past my cerebral palsy and getting to know the real Kerry. Even now we've got our own lives we keep in contact and get together as often as we can. Thanks, girls!

Another brilliant friendship was with three Welsh girls, all with cerebral palsy, who also came to Hereward to find independence and freedom. They knew each other from school and had grown up together. Despite this unique bond,

I was honoured to enter their friendship circle. We hit it off straightaway, giving each other the self-esteem, confidence and drive needed to make the most of college life.

Hereward College was across the road from the local pub, where students often spent their free time enjoying coke and crisps (think not!). The four of us took the chance to get dressed up and go out for a drink! Running late one evening, I arranged to meet them in the pub. An hour later I managed to get halfway to the pub before being confronted with a man lying on the floor with a dog beside him. I really didn't know what to do - it was dark, and I couldn't move. Whichever way I moved, the dog growled and barked. I was stuck, shaking and felt like crying even though it would ruin my make-up. I knew I had to keep calm and not to panic. I didn't want the dog to turn on me. So, thinking quickly, I managed to talk nice and calmly to the dog but shout for HELP!

Eventually, after five minutes which seemed like forever, somebody heard my screams and came to my rescue. An ambulance was called to help the man and I managed to get to the pub! As the man was being treated, his dog bit one of the ambulance crew, trying to protect his owner I suppose.

That was certainly a night to remember. I didn't venture out on my own after that.

As well as enjoying our independence and freedom at Hereward, we achieved a lot of academic success, self-esteem and self-confidence. I got three GCSEs at grades B and C including a B at Tile Hill working alongside Janice and Fiona. I felt ecstatic knowing I achieved a good grade on my own merit.

I wanted to carry on and stretch myself and further my studies. I looked into a BTEC national course in social care at Tile Hill.

This seemed like my ultimate dream come true, especially after having such an amazing year with my GCSEs and meeting Janice and Fiona. But, meeting potential course lecturers, it became clear I was faced with reluctant attitudes. I couldn't believe what I was up against on a course for future social workers and healthcare professionals. I thought I would be an asset and teachers could bounce off my ideas about disability. But the opposition I was faced only made me more determined to get on the course.

I returned home for the summer holidays after my first year at Hereward feeling alone, scared, depressed and a burden as once again I had very few friends in my home town. I relied on family members for my care and social needs. They were the darkest and longest six weeks of my life although I did manage to have my first tattoo and belly button pierced. I wanted to prove to myself I could do such wacky and crazy things! I had to take spasm tablets, but stayed still long enough to get it all done.

I returned to Hereward College in the September for another year of study and adventure. I was on the social care course and determined to work like mad. It was during this year that I met my first boyfriend Chris. I was really excited to know that I could actually meet someone from the opposite sex that I could call my boyfriend. I felt like a normal teenager and I had butterflies in my stomach knowing that somebody was interested in me as more than just a friend. I longed to take it further but I was too scared at the same time. It just felt so right as we had built up a great friendship beforehand and then took it to the next level. I felt so grown up when we announced that we were girlfriend and boyfriend to our friends! It felt so natural, so normal. We had known each other for about a year before our relationship started. We became really close and spent all the time we could together. I was nervous as hell as I didn't have a lot of experience and didn't want to let Chris down. We grew together and our relationship blossomed. I always remember our first kiss. I was worried and scared about going in spasm but Chris gave me a lot of confidence and self- esteem.

The course was a huge challenge, mainly due to negative attitudes and me wanting to prove to everybody I deserved my place. I couldn't believe the hostile attitudes from the lecturers and students alike. On day one students talked over me and above my head and pushed tables and chairs into the back of me on purpose. They even called me a spastic! I couldn't believe it. How could this be happening on a social care course? Despite all the bullying, I found my inner strength to prove people wrong. I ended up calling myself a spastic which eased some of the bullying and helped me to be strong. I was saying 'yes, a spastic can achieve, a spastic can do this course' which inspired me to carry on.

One of the course modules was working with old people and I was placed in a residential home, providing care for elderly residents. My first assignment was to help an Asian lady with her bath routine. As she spoke to me in her own language I didn't understand what she was saying. I called for help as I thought I'd hurt her and to ask my work colleague what she was saying. To my surprise, the lady was praising my capabilities. I was overjoyed, really proud of myself. This gave me a buzz and the confidence I needed to survive and work through the bullying.

The BTEC years were the hardest, loneliest, challenging time but also the most rewarding and soul-searching experience. I learnt to survive and stand up for myself, I learnt to be counted as Kerry. I was no longer patronised or looked down on, I was competing in an able world, being me and surviving.

I successfully came out with top grades. I won't lie, it was fucking hard, fucking horrible. I owed it to myself and others to make it work, make it happen, to survive - and I did survive. I came out with my head held high, a new Kerry, determined to show others I had the right to be counted for me.

On the whole I had a fantastic time at college; college is what you make it, college is what you put into it. We had some amazing adventures and opportunities. I was involved in the production of The Rocky Horror Show. Can you imagine a load of spastics dressed up in stockings, suspenders and basques? It was hilarious, all dressed up and nowhere to go. A drama teacher at Hereward wrote a script of the Rocky Horror Show for students to perform to students, parents and the public. This was adapted from the Rocky Horror film. We all got dressed up in our characters with wicked hair styles and colours to match and acted out the show! After our own production, we went to the Birmingham Hippodrome to watch their performance of the show. It was hilarious. As a bus full of spastics in Rocky Horror costumes, we had a few stares! The only difference was we had wheels and they didn't! We were enjoying ourselves just like everyone else going to the show.

Another wild adventure was the discovery of tattoos! I was 19 when I had my first ever tattoo. After a few Diazepam's my dream came true! To date I have 14! It's true what they say- once you've had one, you can't stop! Over the years, I've managed to find 2 amazing and confident tattooists, one of which has successfully tattooed me 11 times! Absolutely incredible and fantastic. I'm beginning to slow down now because I haven't got much room left on my body! I should really get insured with the amount that it has cost! Each of my tattoos has a story behind them and they are a real credit to the special memories and people in my life. I've even got my favourite poem tattooed on the right-hand side of my body- which stretches from my armpit to my bum!

When someone mentioned university to me, I laughed. I couldn't read or write when I went to special school. Getting GCSEs was amazing, going to college and studying alongside able-bodied students was incredible. Oh, what the heck, let's prove I can go all the way.

Let's get a degree!

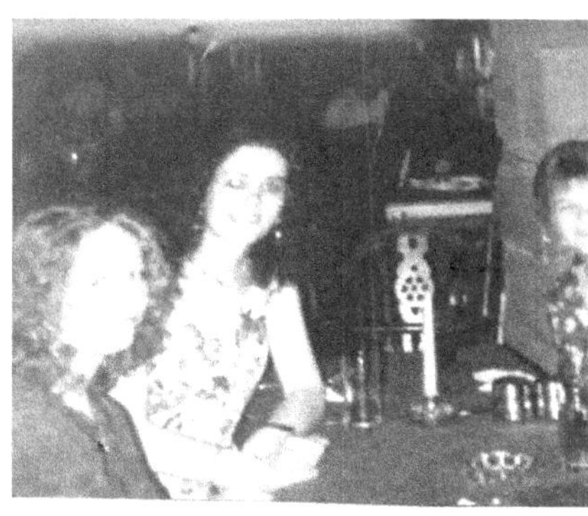

Fiona, Janice and I, aged 18

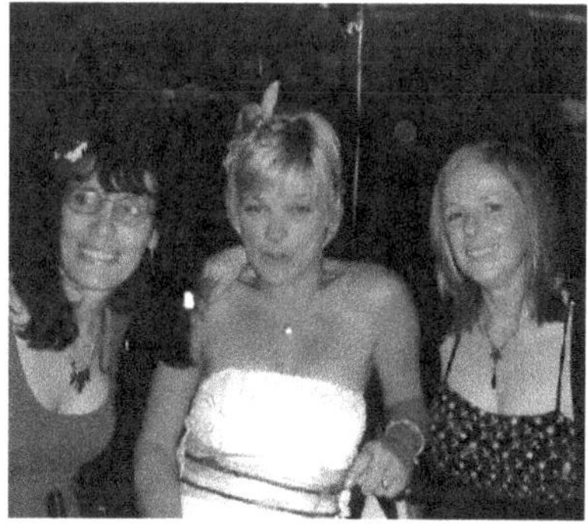

Fiona & Janice at my wedding

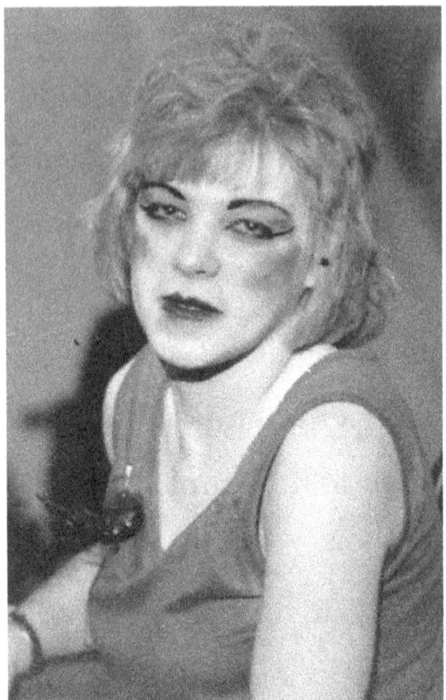

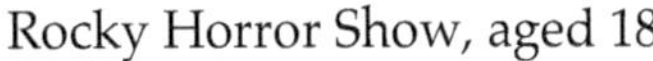

Rocky Horror Show, aged 18

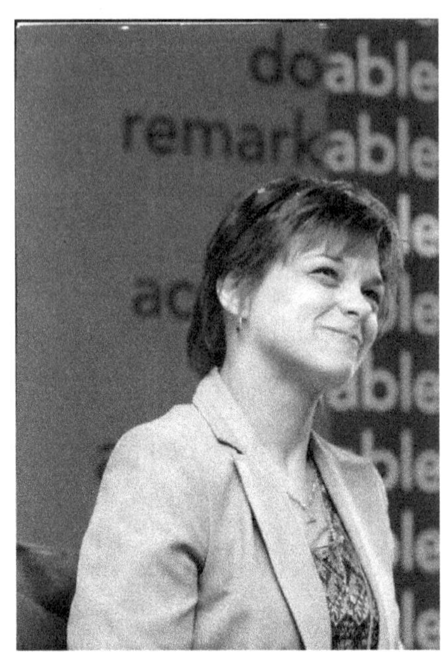

Dublin Conference, aged 25

Sex!

Let's talk about sex baby...
Let's talk about you and me...
Let's talk about all the spasms and CP too...
Let's talk about sex...
All the planning...
All the spasms...
All the fun...
I'm sure we have fun...
With spasms added on too...
Let's talk about sex...

Sex And The Disabled

I'm going to put my hand on my heart and address another taboo subject - sex and the disabled.

I felt really isolated as a teenager as no one explained my body changes and how important this was to becoming a woman. I wanted to be like every other young woman. I wanted to experiment and have my first snog as a teenage girl but, like everything, I had to wait. I couldn't console myself with teenage magazines or gossip in the playground as I didn't have access to either. I was determined that at college I would experiment and find out about normal things like sex.

Hereward College was brilliant, really tuned in to young people with disabilities. Staff knew and understood some of the physical difficulties some students might find having sex with their partner and were trained to assist when needed. My first experience came with my first boyfriend, Chris, at the age of

16. A snog itself was a challenge, let alone anything else! I was so scared of going in spasm and biting his tongue! Luckily, I survived.

Next came the more intimate part of our relationship, sex! Due to the nature of my boyfriend's disability, we were unable to have penetrative sex. We were both young and lacking in experience, but we learnt together and enjoyed experimenting and touching each other's bodies. I was then fortunate enough to meet a French exchange student at Hereward, who gave me my first real sexual encounter. This was a challenge for both of us, as I had to contend with spasms and making sure I didn't spasm at the wrong moment! For him, it was trying to work around my spastic body. We both worked through our own challenges and enjoyed sex together. However, condoms presented a challenge for me, so I left them in his capable hands!

I went on the pill at uni but still made sure my partner wore a condom. After uni, I continued to enjoy experimenting, making sure I was safe and protected whenever I had personal relationships. When I met Chris (not my first boyfriend but I clearly have a fetish for the name Chris… I think it's because a spastic can pronounce it!!), our relationship soon blossomed and, for the first time, I really enjoyed making love to my man. We both had to be creative to make sure we satisfied and pleased each other but this applies to every couple. Sometimes spasms get in the way, other times they enrich the experience.

After 11 years of marriage we still enjoy our occasional intimate time together. I really do hope that my cerebral palsy allows me to enjoy our sex life for many more years to come!

Driving

Who would have thought me driving?
Up and down the motorways
Round and round Spaghetti Junction
Stuck on hills
Pondering with strangers
Such joys
The freedom
The independence
The normality
A spastic in control or
A spastic out of control
You decide!

SPASM
007Z

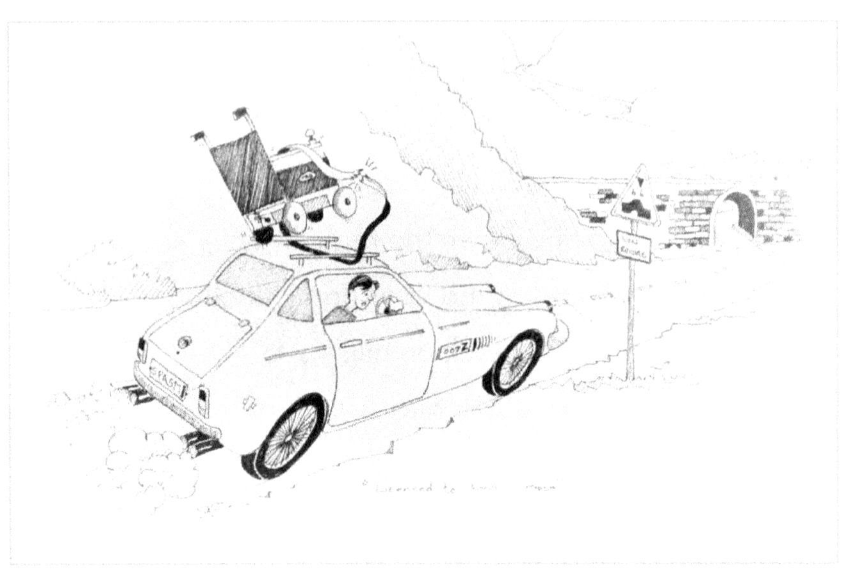

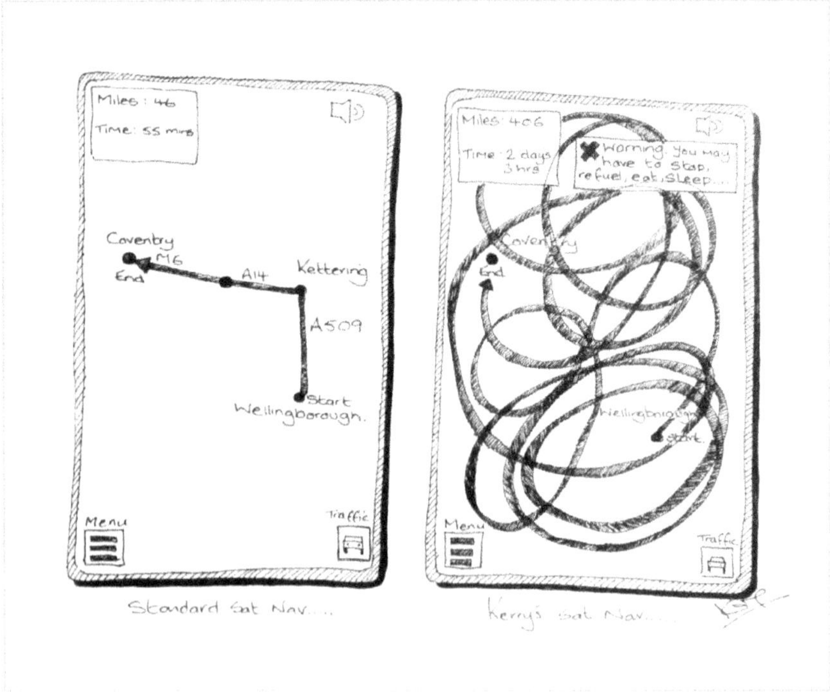
Miles : 46
Time : 55 mins
Coventry
M6
End
A14
Kettering
A509
Start
Wellingborough.
Menu
Traffic
Miles: 406
Time: 2 days
3 hrs
Warning. You may have to stop, refuel, eat, sleep...
Coventry
End
Wellingborough
Start
Menu
Traffic
Standard Sat Nav....
Kerry's Sat Nav....

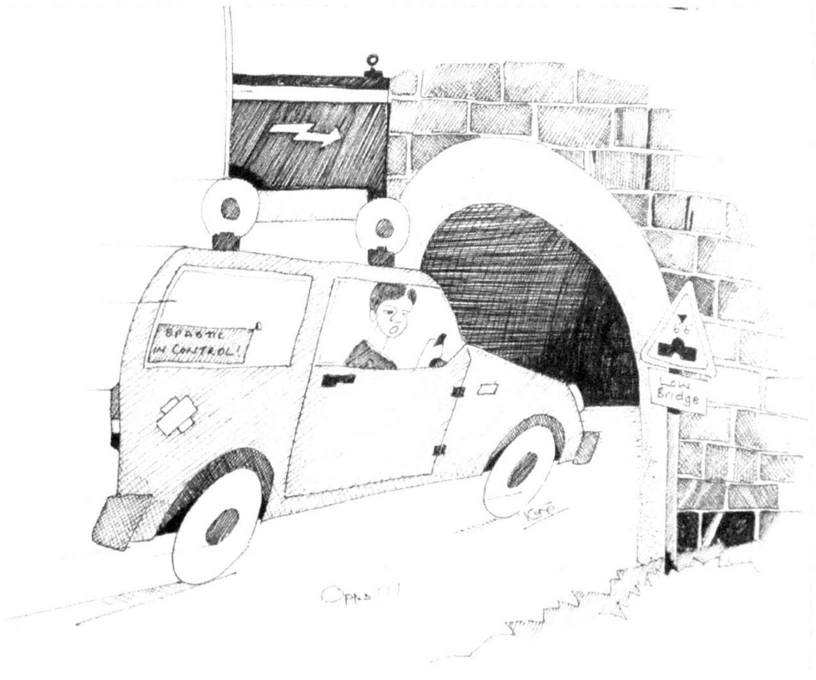

SPASTIC
IN CONTROL!
Low
Bridge
Opps!!!

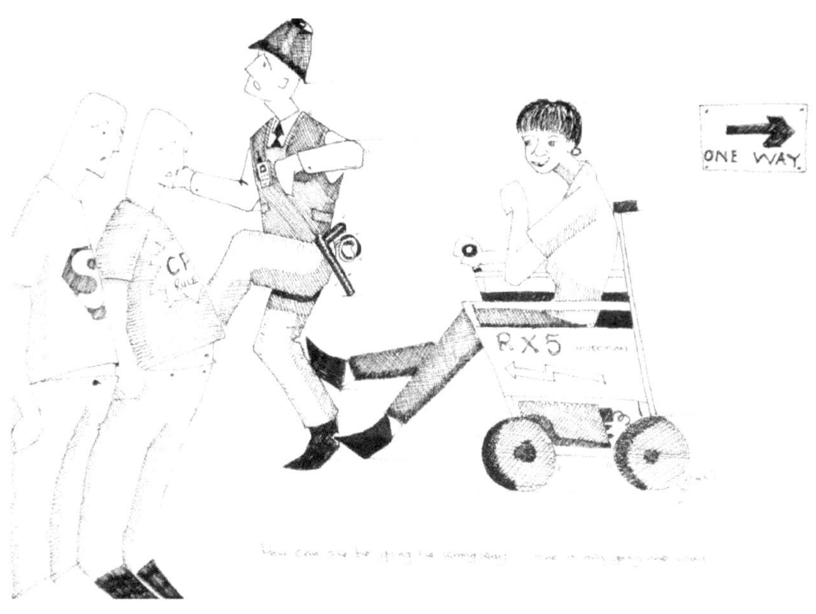
ONE WAY
RX5
CP
Rule

Driving

I still can't believe it even now, but you're beginning to get to know what I'm like. I need to prove them wrong. I get a thought in my head, then look at every possible angle to make it work… driving was no exception.

The subject was first raised when I met Ian (a friend at college with cerebral palsy). His body movements were a lot worse than mine and we got chatting one evening, I asked him what he was waiting for. When his response was – "I'm waiting for my driving lesson" – I was really gobsmacked. I nearly fell out of my chair! Ian had been learning to drive with a local driving school for six months using hand controls. That night I laid in bed and couldn't get driving out of my mind.

This would give me a new lease of life, independence, a sense of normality. I need to prove people wrong, driving I thought was beyond my capabilities. Nothing to lose, everything to gain. It was worth looking into my options. I looked forward to my new challenge although I was scared, anxious and confused just thinking what lay ahead. I decided not to tell many people as I wanted to do my research and find out if it was possible to achieve my dream.

I bumped into Ian again as I thought he would be able to offer advice and answer my questions. He told me about a driving assessment he had to see if he was able to drive. This was organised for me through Hereward College as a group went down to a driving assessment centre for a whole day, which cost in the region of £100, and tested all areas of spatial awareness, hazard assessment, reflexes and understanding the Highway Code. And last, but not least, physical ability. It was an intense, tough day.

I didn't know the result until the end and risked losing £100 and going home disappointed. Passing meant being invited to go on a test drive in an adapted car on a specially designed track. To my amazement, I was able to do my test drive… I was on my way to becoming a driver! I felt normal and able. But how the hell was I going to explain to my family I was going driving?

Reality didn't sink in as I waited six weeks for the paperwork to come before I could start driving lessons. Seemed the longest six weeks ever, but I used the time wisely to find an instructor I felt comfortable with.

When Ian had his next lesson, I asked if I could talk with his instructor and he agreed. John, from Godiva Driving School, was absolutely fantastic from the first time I met him. I felt at ease in his presence. He was the most patient, understanding, sincere person I've ever met, and his sense of humour just came naturally. I managed to rope in two of my friends to learn to drive so John generated a lot of business. The report seemed to take ages to come through but, in all honesty, it wasn't long. I just wanted to get my teeth into it. I passed the report to John, so he was able to follow the guidelines and advice.

It soon became apparent some of the adaptions weren't necessary for my needs, but John worked his way round it. He had the experience and I put all my faith and trust in John. I couldn't sleep the night before my first driving lesson as I was so excited, nervous and anxious. Getting behind the wheel for the first time felt so right, so natural to me. John put me at ease and gave me confidence. We laughed and talked throughout the lesson – there wasn't a moment of silence (little did I know that this was the way to overcome spasms and sudden noises). I felt so normal, so natural and empowered that I was on my way to freedom.

I think the worst challenge was telling my family. I don't think they actually believed I was able to drive until they witnessed it first hand when they came down to see a lesson. It was brilliant, just being free and able. It took 102 lessons before I felt comfortable enough to do my first test, but it didn't matter as this was a challenge I thought was beyond my capabilities. I was really cocky. I told everybody, got a bit big headed and ended up messing it up and failing. I could do everything I'd learnt so naturally, but just messed it up. Looking back, in all honesty, I wasn't used to the silence in the car. On your test you are bound to be nervous, anxious and scared but my spasms took over. I couldn't believe it or understand why, but that night it just clicked: I had no one to talk to.

Now I could understand what John had done. He was blocking out the background noise and it worked. Next day I mentioned it to John and we put theory into practice. Sure enough, with no talking or laughter, I was in spasm, pain and discomfort and losing my concentration. I decided I would talk out loud to myself on my second test to try to alleviate the silence - I knew the examiner couldn't talk back. He might think I was crazy, but anything was worth a try.

I booked my second test and the only person I would tell was John. That really helped loads as I had no pressure, no one to let down. I talked to myself throughout the test. The examiner thought I was losing it! But I didn't care. I talked myself through all the required elements of the test, when I reversed around a corner I knew exactly what I was doing, but still managed to end up on the opposite side of the road! Thankfully as the examiner had heard what I'd been saying he let me complete the task again 10 minutes later. At this time my brain worked with my hands and I finished on the right side of the road!

Talking through things really helped with my jerks, spasms and nerves and at the end of the test the examiner gave me the news I wanted to hear. I was ecstatic. He even apologised for not being able to answer me back when I was having a great conversation with myself!

I was on cloud nine. I had passed my test and I was a driver. My next challenge was to buy my own car. I chose a bright red Peugeot 205 with hand controls. This was my pride and joy and meant everything to me. It was my first new taste of freedom and a new chapter in my life. My family wanted me to have a sticker in my car to make people aware I was a disabled driver. Me being me, I didn't want a disabled sticker, so after thinking long and hard about it, I came up with my own sign. It had a bright red background and white letters saying 'spastic in control'. I found this so liberating and empowering. This was a different opportunity of telling people a spastic can be in control. To me, this was the perfect way to express a positive message and warn other drivers in case I went into spasm.

When volunteering at a local women's hostel I parked in a communal car park to be greeted on my return with a letter on my windscreen from the Unemployed Workers organisation.

They had written their concerns about the sticker being

offensive to people with cerebral palsy! For some people with cerebral palsy it might be, but for me, I see it as a positive, empowering message. They didn't know I had CP. It was highly amusing and, after explaining to them in person the reasons behind my sticker, the matter was resolved very quickly. It was good letter writing practice for them!

I spent many happy years in my car learning ways to overcome obstacles like my spasms and filling up with petrol. One of the most successful ways to alleviate spasm was to keep music on to cut out all the background noise and help me to concentrate. This was put to the test when the CD player broke. I had to drive to Coventry and was once again a nervous wreck, like on my first test. Afterwards I always made sure I had a Wham or Madonna CD to hand.

I enjoyed 10 years of freedom in my car, driving up and down the motorways. It was absolutely phenomenal. I got lost a few times, and once had to have a police escort, but wouldn't change a thing! I remember going to see my first boyfriend at Stoke University. The first weekend I went with a friend and we followed a car in front with no problems at all. We drove from Coventry to Stoke-on-Trent in an hour and a half. So, the second weekend, I decided to brave it myself as I thought I knew what I was doing. Nope!

Coventry to Stoke took six hours… I managed to get myself involved with Birmingham Spaghetti Junction, heading the wrong way on the motorway, filling up with petrol twice and having a police escort! Seriously, I was shitting myself! For those who don't know, Spaghetti Junction is often described, as it says in the title, as spaghetti! There are a lot of intertwining roads all linked to one major road. It's a bit like a maze – once you get in you can't get out! For a first time driver, and if your name's Kerry, it was a total adventure and nightmare! To this day, I don't know how I ended up on it! Never again! On a positive note, it conquered my motorway fears, put it that way! But it was like a bloody fairground ride, going around and round, not being able to get off! Eventually, when I did come off, I was so unbelievably knackered but I strongly believe that allowed me to conquer my fear of motorway driving. I put my life in my hands filling up at a petrol station. I had to trust a complete stranger to do it for me and pay.

I decided to get off and head for a police station as I was

getting really frustrated with going round and round Spaghetti Junction! Enough was enough. Fortunately, I saw a police car and I put my hazards on and they came to my rescue. I must have looked really hassled and panicky and I don't think they could understand my speech (my speech tends to get worse when under pressure or anxious). I really don't think the police could understand what I was saying. I tried to explain where I set off and where I was heading, and I just wanted to get back on the motorway. After about 5 minutes of trying to reassure me and telling me the directions, the police decided that it was somewhat better for them to show me, so they gave me a police escort back to the motorway! To my horror, I was only 20 miles from London... They had put me on the wrong motorway! Still, I managed to conquer my nerves about motorway driving! After that occasion, the journey to Stoke only took an hour.

Another memorable experience was when the three of us decided to go to a McDonalds drive through. You might think that's easy. I think not. Hand controls, three spastics, drink and food weren't a great combination. First, I had to wind down the window and keep my hand on the brake whilst ordering my food. Then I had to pay before working out how to get the food and drinks into the car with a massive queue behind us and the three of us in hysterics! We did it but ended up with a freezing McDonalds...

I spent many happy years driving and exploring many different places, having fun and laughter. I was meeting people from chat rooms, putting my life in danger, being normal... After several years, I began to feel less independent because I couldn't get in the car on my own. I had to rely on different people to help and transfer me. At the time I didn't bat an eyelid but now I can see how dangerous it was.

I needed to explore the possibility of getting in and out of a car and using a wheelchair independently. I started looking at options to make this possible and came up with an adaption for the roof of my car to transport a powered assisted wheelchair to the roof of my Corsa. It was totally phenomenal although the cost was in the region of £10,000. Independence is priceless.

But, after applying to charities and grants, my dream came true. I was totally independent and free, it was amazing. It took me quite a while to get used to the hoist and I had to be careful going under low bridges or up steep hills.

On several occasions I had to call the AA to help me getting the chair from the hoist as it had broken and I was stranded in the car… Looking back, I can see the funny side but, at the time, it was pretty serious.

I relied on my car like everyone else but, once I relocated closer to the town centre, I was hardly using my car at all and, after long and hard soul searching, decided to give up driving. I loved my time driving. I have memorable experiences and adventures. But it seemed the right thing to move forward. I wouldn't change anything. I'm so glad I got talking to Ian when I did. Driving got me to know who the real Kerry is and how determined I am to find a way round things.

I'd be lying to say I don't miss the freedom driving gives such as popping to local shops or going to a friend's house. But, for the times I would use a car, is it really worth it? Life is a challenge going to appointments and meetings etc but, like anyone, you overcome such challenges.

If someone asked me if I'd go back to driving in the future – if you could programme a car without physically having to drive it and I could get in and out without any problems, the answer would be 'yes'. My life is constantly changing and who knows where I will be in five years' time? But, until such technology is available, I'm quite happy relying on an electric wheelchair and public transport.

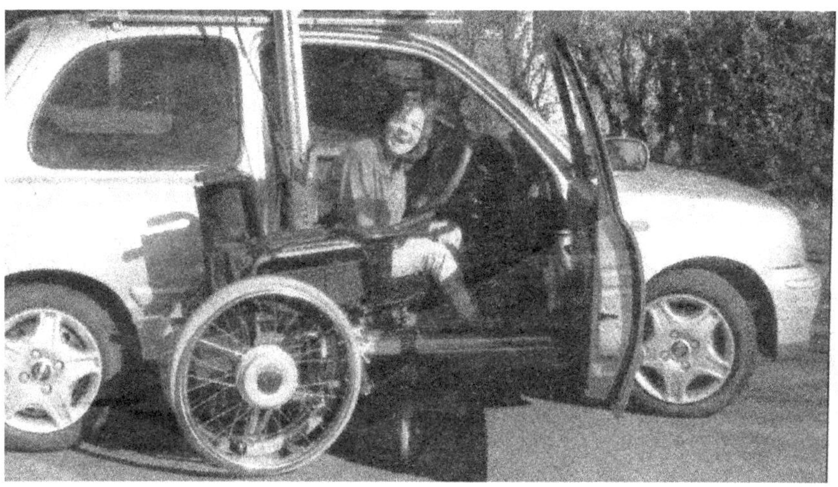

My amazing hoist

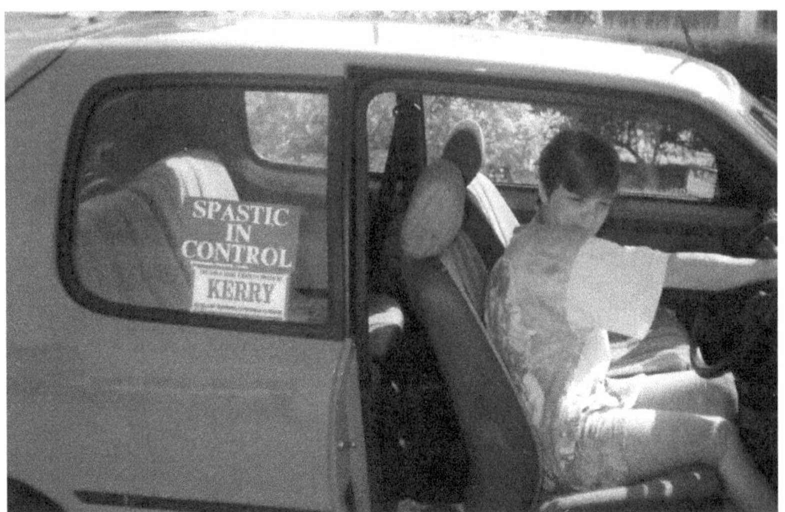

I'm proud of my sticker!

Filming

Stand by… or sit by
Action!
Glamour, glory, make-up
Piss up
Think again!
Nothing like that
Long hours
Take after take
Knackered Boring
Away from home
Pressure
The cost of stardom I was among the stars
I was the star

Esther Marquand eat your heart out!

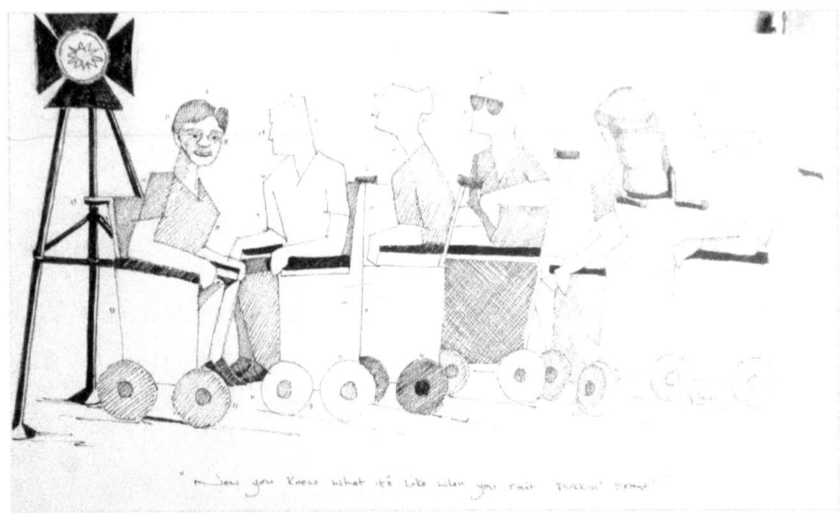

I was just a normal 20-year-old studying at college, minding my own business when stardom struck!

The BBC wanted to adapt Skallagrigg from a book and make it into a film. They wished to use disabled actors rather than able-bodied actors to portray disabled characters. They certainly had a challenge on their hands and, after months of research, decided to come to Hereward College to learn about disability and how individuals cope with their limitations. The principal at Hereward selected a few students to talk to researchers about disability.

On the day of the meeting I was more concerned about having the whole day off from the bullying I was receiving doing my BTEC at Tile Hill. I decided to meet the researchers and see what happened. A screen test would enable the director and producer to make an informed decision. Once the test was set up, everybody in the room started acting really silly and I genuinely felt embarrassed for the researcher. I honestly thought he was researching disability and didn't realise the full consequences of my actions!

I was learning to drive, so decided to go ahead and talk about driving. I was gabbing away not realising the impact I was having! Afterwards I went back to my studies and forgot about the researchers. The following week the principal asked if I remembered what I had done. I thought I was in trouble but then he told me the producer, director and writer had seen my clip from the audition and wanted to come down to meet with me. Still unaware of my actions and how such a major experience would take me, I agreed to meet with them.

The following week I auditioned for the main role in Skallagrigg as Esther. I would be playing a teenage girl with cerebral palsy in a quest to find The Skallagrigg. Esther had severe cerebral palsy and the producer and director wanted to make my speech deliberately worse in order to trick the audience, making them believe they were really understanding what Esther was saying.

I could see thumbs going up and nods being made. I thought this was a positive sign and carried on!

Again I returned to my studies and genuinely forgot about my second audition. The following week I received another visit asking me if I wanted the part of Esther in the film and to complete the necessary course work before embarking on a filming career! This was sheer madness, not in my plans at all. But it was an opportunity of a lifetime and I decided to grab it with both hands and see where the adventure would take me. My first challenge was to tell my course leader. This was more problematic than I first thought. She gave me three weeks to finish my course work before filming. She didn't know but I'd already been working my socks off, the course work was handed in before the allocated time! I was very determined not to let this opportunity slip through my fingers.

I was invited to London for more auditions and to meet the

cast. Arriving at the BBC studios I was absolutely shell shocked, being led through the corridors, looking at all the photos on the walls of famous people. I couldn't believe it! I was led into a room of around 50 other people, some in wheelchairs but mostly able-bodied. I was introduced to a few people but couldn't remember their names or who they were. These included Bernard Hill, Kevin Wheatley, Ian Dury and Richard Briars. The read through went really well and I started to understand more about the film and the character I was about to take on.

It was decided to visit Madame Tussauds in our characters to spend the day getting to know our roles. Bernard Hill was going to take the role of my dad in the film, so we had to build up an onscreen relationship as father and daughter. I found this a real challenge and very thought provoking as I had to win Bernard over as well as get to know him and his character. Like everything, I love challenges! If I put my mind to something and I believe in what I am doing, then I will achieve my aim.

The day at Madame Tussauds went extremely well. I forgot a few times that I was in character and that my name was

Esther and not Kerry. This confused me a little, but I soon adapted to being Esther. After a week at The Kensington Hilton in London, living the highlife of ordering burger and chips through room service and charging it to the BBC's bill, it was time to hit the road and Esther to be born.

My filming would last for eight weeks, with 12-hour working days and only five days off during that time. When the contract came through, it was all-too-easy not to read the small print as filming seemed fun, exciting and glamorous. How wrong could I be! I didn't realise the full impact of filming and the implications it would have on me and my cerebral palsy. To be fair none of the disabled actors did. Filming was long with little time to ourselves. There was lots of travelling and staying in different hotels.

I was doing 12 hours a day, six days a week, and that in itself caused me spasms. Add the fact you film scenes out of sequence and had to keep track what stage your character is at, it was really hard work, especially in all kinds of weather with CP and spasms to contend with. I now appreciate why films don't have disabled actors in them.

I always remember my first fuck up. I'd been working two weeks solid and travelled to three different locations. I was freezing cold but, as we were filming out of sequence, I was made to wear jeans and a t shirt without a coat. I didn't understand fully about continuity because I was tired, cold and in spasm. It took longer to film and I really fucked up big time. Everyone was putting immense pressure on me and I told the director what he could do with his film! He said that the scene 'would not cut together well', due to continuity and spasms. I told him to stick his film and if he wanted an able-bodied actress, he should have got one! Bernard Hill and the others backed me all the way. Later that night I got to watch my first takes and began to see why we had to film so many takes.

Filming was fucking hard work, demanding and soul searching but, at the same time, I met some amazing people and we formed a family, working and living together. I changed a lot of preconceived attitudes surrounding disability and CP, for the better, I hope! Once we had finished filming Skallagrigg, I returned to college and continued with my BTEC, obtaining top grades, almost forgetting I'd been involved with a film.

A year after the filming, I was involved in voice overs and piecing together the film. It's incredible to think a film can take a year to make from start to finish. The voice overs were incredibly hard, especially when you add CP into the equation! Your mouth doesn't always coordinate with your spasms, making it impossible to achieve such a thing. Once again, I had a heated debate with the producer and director allowing them to appreciate my point! We did successfully achieve voiceovers that both parties were happy with.

When Skallagrigg was launched, I was involved in publicity. My name was in all the TV magazines! It was surreal, something you would only dream of. I did several interviews alongside Bernard Hill including a live chat on Pebble Mill at One with Ross King. I took two of my friends from college to sit in the audience. I decided I would walk on to the set with the help of Bernard. During the interview, I experienced a lot of spasms, but Bernard came to the rescue and knew exactly what to do. I had taught him how to restrain my spasm attacks and how to put pressure on the muscles. I suppose it looked funny but Bernard was totally brilliant.

The launch itself was incredible as I got to see the film for the first time in London. I felt so honoured, excited, nervous and happy. Seeing my name as a second credit made me cry.. After all the hard work, pain, spasm, tears and laughter, everything seemed so right.

Shortly after the film was screened, I received several pieces of fan mail, one even asking for my autograph! I couldn't believe it; I was star struck. I'm so glad I had this amazing opportunity with Bernard playing my dad, I managed to win him over and change his views on disability.

A year later I was approached by the British Film School who were producing a short film for their end-of-year assessment called 'A Long Way Home'. As it was a student film, the budget was really low and wasn't on such a huge scale. I helped them out by becoming involved in their production and, in return, they hired an electric wheelchair for me which somehow survived a three-year stint with me at university! Looking back, if asked to do another bloody film now, I'd say, "No way, I love my bed too much!"

Aim your goals high
And you will achieve
Aim your goals low
And you won't achieve
You will feel high if you achieve
So go and set yourself a goal
And
ACHIEVE

University

It's time to fly the nest Let the adventure begin
For many this is a fun and exciting time Leaving home and standing on your own two feet Not for me
Scary Fear
Have I bitten off more than I can chew?
Who will help?
Who will support me?
All the normal questions a student would ask But I'm a spastic!
I shouldn't have come this far
I shouldn't have been able to write my own name Let alone GCSEs and A levels

A degree
Me, Kerry, first in the family When people say I can't
Kerry says she does and she will Fun times
Highs Lows
Drunken days Drunken nights
A lot of hard slog And a lot of Botox too But you know what?
I wouldn't change a thing

That standing ovation at my graduation
Meant the world to me
And I can hold my head up high
With my 2:1 Honours Degree in Sociology And Women's
Studies
You know what?
A spastic can achieve
A spastic can make anything they want
Out of life
So what's that word again?
You CAN do it You CAN do it!

I was on my adventures yet again! This time a big challenge, something I never thought would happen in my wildest dreams. But, once I make my mind up, I always achieve my dreams no matter what! This would be no exception.

I'm off to university! I managed to secure a place at five different universities, which was amazing. One uni offered me an unconditional place without even meeting me. Once arriving there, it was clear they hadn't studied the final details of my application form, especially the disabled part! Ah well, at least I got offered a place on my own merit, not because I was disabled.

I took the easier option of going to a uni that already had disabled students. I really didn't want to be another guinea pig after my college years. Uni was going to be a big enough challenge for a disabled student. Staffordshire Uni (Stoke-on-Trent site) offered the right course, wasn't that far from home and Alton Towers was just around the corner! The uni had a great policy and reputation for disabled students, organising support needs and making sure disabilities weren't the main focus.

After several meetings with the disability department, it was decided I would have a full-time live-in support worker funded by my local authority and live on campus in a shared house with another disabled student and their support worker. So far so good, brilliant. My support package was sorted, all I had to do was concentrate on being a student!

The day finally arrived. I was going to uni to study a degree in Sociology and Woman's Studies. I couldn't believe what I was doing. I packed my bags, equipped with dungarees, Doc Martens and a stock of loo paper! Off I set in my car to uni.

People didn't know what was about to hit them but would soon find out!

I was determined to live uni life to the full and not let anything stand in my way. I knew it was going to be difficult and frustrating but was determined to survive. Couldn't let this opportunity slip through my fingers without a fight! I felt nervous, scared, anxious and apprehensive about being a spastic at uni but these thoughts were overridden by feelings of excitement, empowerment and enthusiasm.

After driving from my hometown to Stoke in my loaded car, I arrived at my shared house, my home for three years. I was really excited to be greeted by my two male housemates, Pete and Nigel. They seemed a little reluctant to be moving into a house equipped for disabled students, but I soon put them at ease, and we hit it off laughing and joking. Neither knew much about disability but, as mature students, were eager to learn.

Ours was two houses knocked into one and had ten bedrooms, three bathrooms and two kitchens. I shared the ground floor with another disabled student in her third year and her support worker. Upstairs was occupied by other first year male and female students. During the first week we all got to know each other really well and helped whenever and however we could. It soon became apparent I needed a lot more support than one support worker. I decided to use them mainly for my academic studies as opposed to my 'care needs'.

I was very independent and needed minimal help with dressing and cooking. The way I worked around this scenario was like this: I had a car and students needed to go shopping;

I needed my shoes on. Housemates put my shoes on in return for a lift to the local shops! This was a brilliant set up for me to achieve my goals without really acknowledging my disability.

Uni life was fantastic; like a "normal" student, I got up in the morning, showered, dressed, got someone to put my shoes on and went to lectures, then returned home to study! I always knew I had to study harder than my able-bodied peers due to my disabilities. I couldn't afford to leave assignments to the last minute, always having to keep on top and be well organised.

Once my study day was over, it was time for something to eat, I was determined to have as little support from my friends as possible. I wanted to see how much I could do for myself and was determined to push the boundaries! One night I cooked fish fingers, chips and beans. Sounds simple but, think again, I was a spastic having to cook on the floor. First challenge was clearing a space! Students' kitchens weren't the best and washing up needed to be done beforehand. The kitchen wasn't the cleanest; it would probably have been better to buy new cutlery. But I was highly determined to cook.

I had the best fish fingers, chips and beans ever. Despite it being cold, I enjoyed every mouthful. I got some help with the washing up, leaving it on the side to show people Kerry meant business!

That night I went to the Students' Union, as usual, determined to have a good time and be a student. I wanted to wear some new earrings and was struggling to get my shoes on. As the other students had gone out, I decided to go next door and ask for help. After banging on a few doors, I ended up going to a house four doors away. I went back to my house to fetch my stuff and found the door shut. I had forgotten my key! Had to wait a bloody hour until someone came back and let me in! Oh, it was fun! Still had a really good night though.

I always went out to the Students' Union across the road from my house on my own, but I never seemed alone. It was brilliant. I was on an equal footing with able-bodied students. I felt able and strong competing with everyone. I made some great friends who took me for Kerry as we supported each other through the highs and lows of uni. Helen was 19 years old and, like most, away from home for the first time. She had a twin sister at another uni and was missing her like crazy. We became really good friends, supporting each other in times of need. Helen offered me physical support, and, in return, I gave her some emotional support. We worked really well as a team.

I remember one particular night at the Students' Union bar. I was getting a drink with other students watching. It soon became obvious to them that disabled students got served quicker. During the evening I pulled this fit bloke and we had a few dances, with me out of my wheelchair. When I went back to get my wheelchair it had gone! Shit, how was I going to get this bloke back to mine? I discovered my wheelchair had been taken by one of my friends so he could get served quicker at the bar. Fair play to him! My wheelchair came in handy for helping me get a few good snogs and quicker drinks for my friends!

I admit I overdid it in the first year. Every student does but, for me, this had a detrimental effect. It sounds strange but I forgot about my disability. I just wanted to enjoy uni life and the freedom it brought. I was discovering who Kerry was and I loved it. I was living an able-bodied life in a spastic body. How long could this last?

Not long....my body gave me warning signs I failed to acknowledge. I was having such a good time. Then crunch! One day I got up as normal to do my usual routine and my body wouldn't follow my brain. I had a few spasms, as normal, but this time they lasted and lasted. Eventually I was in spasm for 22 hours a day. On one occasion my hands reached my head and I went into spasm and pulled great chunks out of my hair. It was so scary, frightening and horrible. I didn't know what to do, my whole world was crumbling around me...

This went on for two whole weeks. Finally, Pete and Nigel decided enough was enough and took me to casualty. The doctors administered a diazepam drip. This was absolutely brilliant until the effects wore off and I was back in crippling muscle spasm. I couldn't believe what was happening and was forced to return home to sort myself out! All my friends at uni were fantastic and continued to go to lectures and write notes for me. After six weeks at home, I was well enough to go back to uni to continue my first year of study. I successfully completed my course work a month after the due date and exams for the year within the allocated time. I was really proud of myself.

I spoke with specialists and decided to sign up for the Botox trial for people with cerebral palsy at Stoke. Trials were incredibly difficult, injections were administered in front of about 20 doctors, which in turn led to increased spasm and high muscle tone. It was extremely painful and distressing. The reward came two weeks after receiving the injections when I successfully took my first independent steps. It felt amazing until I laughed and fell over! The doctor said: "If you hadn't laughed, you would be walking!" My response was that, if I hadn't laughed, it wouldn't be me!

I was 22 years old and finishing my degree outweighed the importance of walking. I was born with CP and I will die with it. The Botox alleviated the pain and spasm I was having and allowed me to live life to the full and that's what matters to me. I calmed down socialising a bit in my second year and listened to my body. This was really hard when competing with able-bodied students but having such an amazingly supportive network of friends really helped. Year two was much harder than the first but I successfully gained a 2:1 grade, which I was extremely proud of. I had learnt my lesson the hard way from my first year…

As with most students, my third year was extremely difficult but, as always, I rose to the challenge and started my dissertation early. I chose to research women with disabilities who had attended special education in my home town. I chose this study as it meant I could conduct the research over the summer holidays and it certainly paid off!

I managed to rope a good friend of mine, Elaine, into escorting me to the people's homes to conduct interviews with young disabled women. Elaine was brilliant. We had grown up together and known each other since we were 10 years old. She lived in the same neighbourhood, on my street. Once again, my disability was no issue to Elaine – she would just get on with it. We went on crazy nights out and holidays, and we'd been there for each other through thick and thin.

When I returned to Stoke, I opted out of the support package from the uni and organised my support myself. This was really successful as I used a local care agency, as well as students who had graduated the year before. I really enjoyed my third year at uni and, despite the hard work, continued to socialise with my friends. As a result of my dedication and willpower, I was awarded a 2:1 BA Honours degree in Sociology and Women's Studies. At my graduation I received a standing ovation; I felt so humbled and touched by this.

University gave me definitely the most challenging, soul searching, thought provoking years of my life so far. I was so glad I was able to have this experience and truly believe I made the best of the opportunities and experiences on offer.

Since 1997 I have worked with a number of different support workers to enable me to live an independent lifestyle. I started life after uni having 24 hour care, at the time this was very difficult to accept and appreciate, as I consider myself very independent. "An able mind and a spastic body". After uni I flat shared with a friend from uni, this was great for the first 6 months but then she became homesick and returned back to her home town. Over those 6 months we learnt together how to run a house, budget, and do all the necessary things. I then employed an agency to provide my 24 hour support. Again, this aided my independence but I hated the fact that a complete stranger turned up on my doorstep once a week and then stayed the whole week... I met some incredible and amazing people over the years from all different walks of life. I can share a story or two about most of them!

Zoe was one of my 24 hour support workers in the early days and she was incredible. She was shy, naïve and gullible. We made a great team, learnt together, and conquered many things. She stayed with me for a week or two weeks at a time, with a week off. We learnt to cook, clean, party and make home. Thanks Zoe for the great learning curve.

Over the years I've learnt to survive without 24 hour care, and have had numerous support workers, good and bad. Some wanted to take over, not understanding it or appreciating my independence, just judging my body before my mind, and believe me I soon showed them where the door was!

One of the key ingredients of being my support worker is letting me make my own "fuck ups" and just acting as my hands and appreciating it's my life. One such person is Simone Harvey, who has survived an incredible 8 years to date! She just gets me. She knows when to step back and step in. She's become a member of the family.

My care package now is brilliant, I've got a great team who really appreciate my need to be independent, and they know when to step in and step out and be my hands not my brain…

Thanks guys… you know who you are. What a great team we are. You just get me. I wouldn't know what to do without you.

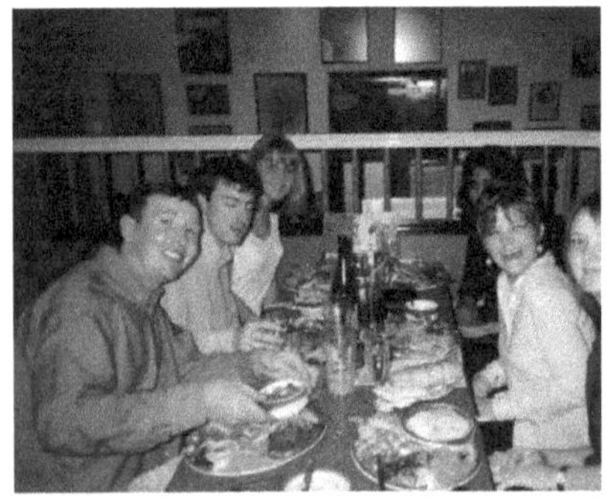

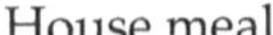

House meal

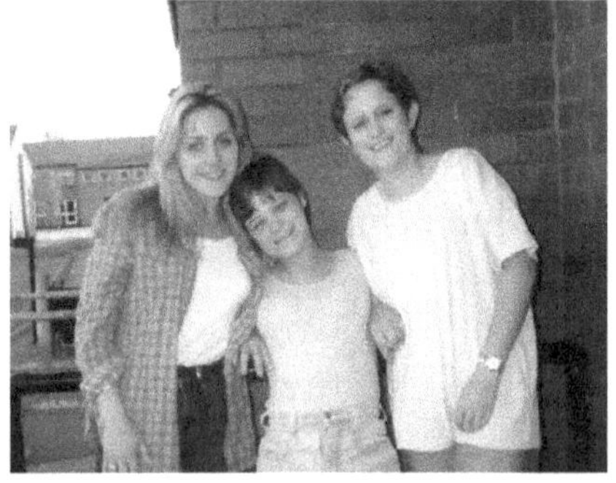

Helen and Marie, first year of uni

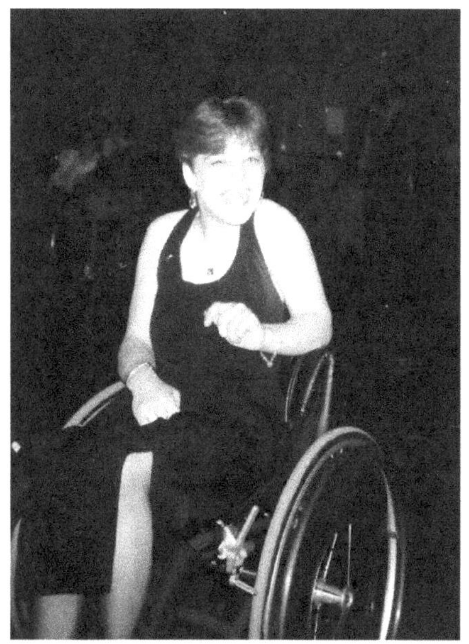

My 21st birthday at uni

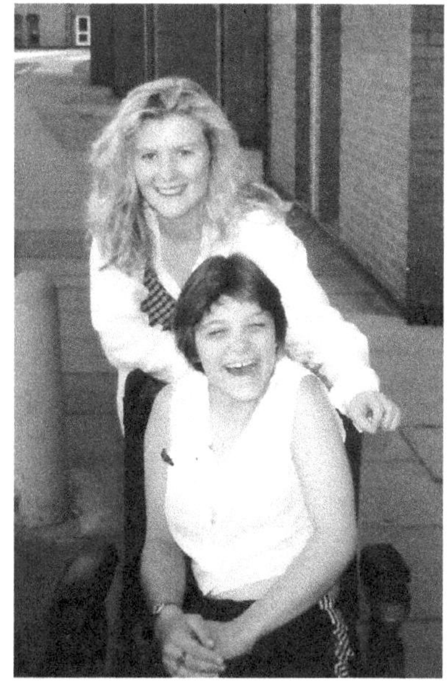

Me and Emma at uni

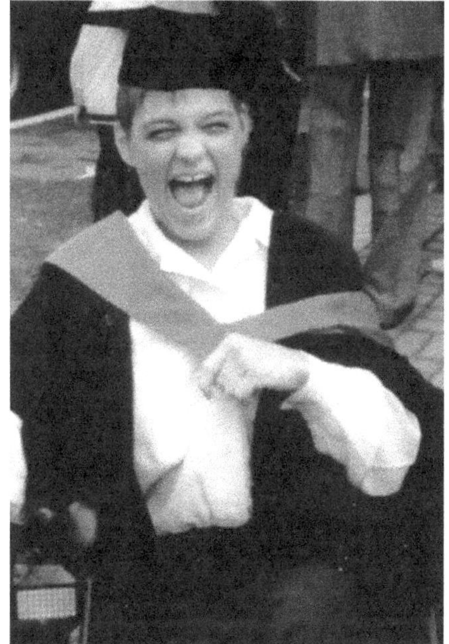

My Graduation

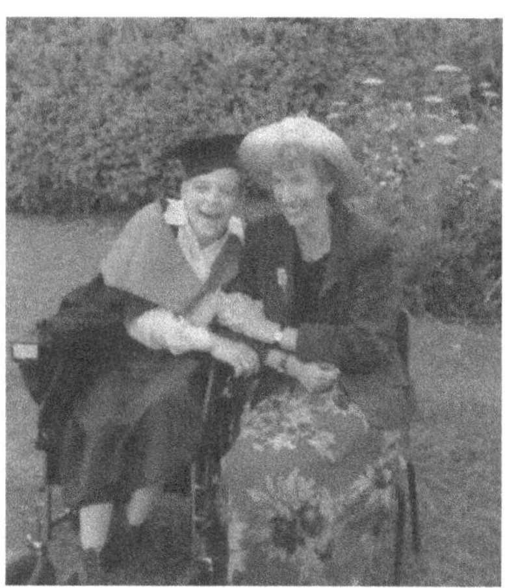

Me and Leah at my Graduation

Snowy, Simba And Tia Maria

A graduate!
Brill
Reality
Oh God!
A job
A home
I can do it
Or can I?
I've got this far on my own
Why not go further?
I'm independent
Or am I?
The things I can't do
Putting shoes and socks on
Getting in and out of the car
It's a nightmare now
What do I do?
I should be happy
I'm a graduate!
But instead
I'm stuck in a rut...

Independence or Not

Is this independence?
What is independence?
An independent mind
Or an independent body
I've got one
But not the other…

I can do most things
With sure determination

But the little things I can't seem to conquer
Shoelaces
Making tea
Putting earrings in
Shaving armpits and legs!...
But all this adds up to independence…

I found myself at a dead end and at probably the darkest point in my life so far… It should have been the happiest, exciting and most challenging time. I was only 24 and had already been through hell and back in all kinds of ways with my disability, and now I felt I was being punished for who I was and standing up for myself.

I often feel like there are two groups of disabled people. My school mates mostly sat back after we left and let everyone do everything for them. They achieved little in the way of independence. Others become disabled later in life and believe the world owes them a living. Talk to them and they'll jump down your throat, because they know what it's like to be able-bodied and the attitudes that they receive.

Then there was little old me, 24 years old, wondering what the hell to do next. I thought going to uni would be the answer to all my dreams and aspirations. Wrong. Yes, I had my own front door but was far from independent. I felt like I'd been dumped here and forced to have 24-hour care. I hated having to rely on people to put my shoes and socks on, make dinner, clean the house, do the laundry, help me to my car. I felt trapped inside my home.

I wanted to be back at uni where I was strong and independent. There I could get out and about and be the same as everybody else. Students, in general, rely on each other and I wasn't any different. I was probably in a better position than many as I had a car and that's how I managed my care needs, (you do this for me and I will take you shopping in the car). Life seemed so simple; suppose it was really, that's university for you, a different world. Every student goes through a period of adjustment after uni to get integrated back into the world.

I'd just graduated from uni with a 2:1 honours degree in Sociology and Women's Studies. I should have been on cloud nine, planning my future, mapping my life out in front of my eyes and to be fair it was like that for the best part of six months. I was happy, content and secure yet missing the real Kerry, the fun loving, enthusiastic, get-up-and-go Kerry I was at uni. I felt isolated, trapped, lonely and confused. Was this independent living?

I found myself getting up in the middle of the night to turn the carer's tele off while they were tucked up in bed. It was crap; they didn't even hear me calling for help. Life seemed to be going backwards. I should have been able to strive towards my goals and dreams just like a normal graduate. Enough was enough; the only way to change the situation was grab hold of life with both hands and stand up for myself and get back to being Kerry! I needed a purpose. But how?

I needed someone to depend on me. Kids? Pets? Job? Kids were out of the question as I didn't even have a partner!

Second on the list was pets. I decided to have an indoor rabbit, yes a rabbit! The garden centre saw me coming! Gave me a big list of things I'd need before I bought the rabbit. Yes, gullible Kerry bought everything and more and it cost me a fortune!

I really hoped "Snowy" would give me the company and companionship I craved. He was cute, a little bundle of white fluffy cotton wool with a pink button nose which twitched as he hopped about. I loved Snowy and was determined to handle him as much as possible. However, one day whilst holding Snowy, I went into spasm and squeezed the poor little mite. He didn't half squeal. I felt awful. Sadly, Snowy died soon after.

Later I learnt rabbits can have heart attacks when they have a sudden shock. I really loved that rabbit to bits!

After a few months feeling at a loss, I decided to try again with another pet. This time a cat (I must admit as a child I hated cats as they made me jump and go into spasm!). So, God only knows why I chose a cat! A friend had a cat that ran up the curtains and, then halfway across the pelmet, suddenly jump down on top of me. This didn't help my spasms. So why a cat?!...

Driving towards Cambridge, I saw a sign to Wood Green Animal Shelter and turned in to have a look round. I had a mental list of what I wanted out of a cat, thinking it would never really come true, as I would not find all my 'wants' in one cat.

The list somewhat went like this......indoor cat for selfish reasons; doesn't jump too much (due to spasms) and likes lots of fuss and attention.

Chances are you would never find that in one cat, or could you?

To my shock and disbelief, a cat brought in the previous day ticked all the right boxes. Simba had been abused and mistreated by his previous owners and needed to be an indoor cat for his own safety.

When I heard Simba's story, I fell in love with him straightaway and knew our bond would be strong. Together we learnt to build up trust. The bond we had was brilliant and he gave me so much joy and confidence. I learnt to live again. I felt happy and content but however after a while I began to sink into my old habits of feeling down, confused and lonely. I hated having to rely on 24-hour care to make my life spontaneous. Carers who didn't know me turned up at my flat and stayed for a week or maybe two. However I still needed to get out and about so had to accept the situation, simple as that, right?

So, nothing kept me down for long! I decided to seek a volunteering role at a special school in Northamptonshire that catered for children with Cerebral Palsy and such disabilities. Here I enabled young children with Cerebral Palsy to meet an older person with a similar physical disability to them. This enabled them to appreciate and understand that their disability is for life and to gain a positive role model for them to be inspired by. Throughout this time, I met some incredible teachers and support workers. One of which was Jan Hall (the music therapist). We instantly clicked and shared a similar quirky sense of humour. Jan lived in my home town and we often shared a few nights out and she became a great friend of mine- always seeing past my disability and enabling me to live my life to the full.

Where was I? Oh yeah, a job! It's every graduate's dream to secure their first job, so why should I be any different? But I am a spastic and my name's Kerry! So, yes, I am different! I applied for different jobs but had the qualifications without the experience. So I decided to work at a local disabled charity which supported people with physical disabilities often lacking the confidence or skills to speak for themselves. I was an intermediary or advocate for them. I acted as a "voice" in meetings and/or appointments offering them self-esteem and confidence either to speak for themselves or stepping in when needed to let their voice be heard. This was extremely empowering for both parties as it allowed me to give that individual the self-esteem they needed in their lives and in return I gained tremendous job satisfaction knowing that I gave something back that comes so natural to me.

I really loved my new challenge and gained valuable experience enabling other disabled people to achieve their goals and aspirations. After doing work experience, the charity offered me a job as a mentor with a salary of £12k a year – a good salary for a graduate in the mid-1990s. Every graduate's dream, yippee! Things were looking up; I was so excited I couldn't believe it. I was back to being the old Kerry again. I felt I could prove to myself and others I was entitled to be in an able-bodied world and survive. This was my ideal first job inspiring people with learning disabilities to lead a fulfilling life. My self-esteem had just doubled. This was the best news ever since graduating. I had begun to think I'd made the worst decision of my life going back to my hometown after uni. Now things were looking up....

Then my bubble burst. I was told I couldn't accept the job due to the cost of my care needs. It would have cost me more than half my wages just getting to work. It was really stupid. I knew I could do the job and was so pissed off and confused and lonely. I still had my Simba (and I wouldn't squeeze him to death, lesson learnt the hard way!). But I couldn't really centre my world on him.

After this disappointment, life was pretty grim and I found myself in a downward spiral. I hated where I was. I was at my darkest time and felt really vulnerable. I needed to get out and find myself again. I was bored, a burden, trapped, frustrated, with no direction in my life. Driving to get cat litter for Simba, I found myself going back to the animal shelter. There I fell in love again with a beautiful eight-week-old abandoned kitten.

The runt of the litter, nobody wanted her. Her three brothers had been rehomed together, but she was left behind. After hearing her story, I knew I needed to take her home and love her. Her fur was a mix of browns and blacks and she walked with an air of her own importance.

Tia Maria won my heart and joined my family! I wasn't sure what Simba thought of the new arrival, but they lived together happily for many years.

Chatrooms

I'm bored.......
I'm lonely......
I'm confused
I need to meet people
I need to be me
I need to be free
I need to get out more
I can't.......
I'm stuck......
I wish I was back at uni
But I'm not....
What can I do?
Are chatrooms the answer?
At least I can be the real Kerry.....

Don't know what possessed me to do it but one night I got totally fed up and turned to my computer. I found myself entering the world of chatrooms. At first, I didn't know what I was doing as I was new to this form of Internet. It felt exciting waking up in the middle of the night wanting to go back to the chatroom.

I could pretend I was someone else. I was back to the old Kerry. These people didn't know I was spastic, they didn't know me from Adam. It was a release from 24-hour care, things I couldn't do, from reality. It felt normal, like being back at uni. I was no longer seen as Kerry who couldn't do anything. I was Kerry who had just graduated from uni and enjoyed life.

I could tell people what I wanted instead of them making judgements around my cerebral palsy. There was a sense of excitement forming friendships in chatrooms. I found myself waiting to go back on and chat to my new social outlet of friends. Over a period of months, I got braver and started flirting with guys in the chatroom. It felt normal and exciting. I didn't worry about the other side. If I wasn't telling the truth about who I was, who were they? Didn't matter. I wouldn't be rejected. I loved it. I was free.

Reality hit home when the telephone bill dropped through the door. Oh my God, my addiction had cost me a fortune. I had to tackle this head on. I had a dilemma. I had formed 'real' friendships I didn't want to say goodbye to but must cut down the phone bill. So I gave my number to several people who lived fairly locally and stayed in contact. I was full of excitement waiting for the phone to bleep when a message came through.

After several months communicating this way I took the plunge to meet. Looking back, I was bloody stupid and naïve but didn't give a shit. I just wanted to meet people. I was lonely but felt loved by my 'new friends'. I decided to meet a guy in the next town keeping my home address secret. I asked him before we met to help me out the car so I could go on my own and be independent. I knew I shouldn't have done but I just wanted to be myself. Anyway, he turned up and seemed a lovely guy. He got me out of the car, we went for a drink and had a great afternoon.

After our 'date', I asked him to put me back in the car, which he did. Then he opened his heart to me – he had a hidden disability. I thought he was going to say epilepsy or hearing problems, something on those lines…. but, no, he claimed he was schizophrenic and turned really nasty, ranting and randomly shouting abuse to me. He was really insistent he wanted to come home with me. Thinking quickly, I decided to let him follow me in his car to my home. This might sound stupid but at least I was able to get back in my car. Halfway home, I indicated right at a roundabout and made sure he turned right before carrying on straight ahead! I nearly caused an accident, but it was better than what could have happened. Back home, I received a lot of abusive texts and phone calls. In the end I had to change my number. I couldn't believe how stupid I had been. Several months later I decided to steer clear of chatrooms and keep safe.

Next I tried the lonely hearts column in Disability Now magazine. I edged toward an advert asking for a companion in a similar situation to myself and receiving 24-hour care. We got chatting and writing and eventually arranged to meet up.

However, we both had different views and outlooks on life.

For example, I'm a strong believer that, if you can do it yourself no matter how long it takes, you should do it! From an early age, kids with CP are encouraged to do things themselves and you should carry that on throughout adulthood. I don't know what it's like to do things in five minutes, but I know me and I get great satisfaction knowing I achieved that goal on my own. I've had cerebral palsy all my life, why should it be any different now I'm in my twenties? However, this guy didn't follow my views and we both decided not to pursue the relationship anymore!

I went back into chatrooms, but this time wasn't as naïve and had managed to sort myself out a better deal on the Internet. After several months, I was ready to meet up again, but this time I made sure I wasn't on my own. I came across a fun-loving bloke in his late twenties with a spinal injury. We got talking on the net and later arranged to meet up. We had lots in common and our relationship blossomed. Soon we were spending weekends and holidays together, just enjoying each other's company. However, it became apparent distance was hindering our relationship. I lived in Northamptonshire and he was in Loughborough. So I decided to uproot and move to Loughborough. The whole process took over a year to complete. During that time, we managed to enjoy our relationship, going away at weekends and holidays and having fun. I found myself living for weekends and holidays!

I still felt really isolated and low about my daily life; I'd found love, but my life felt empty. I needed to find out why I was beating myself up inside. I couldn't just live for weekends and holidays and wait to start my new life in Loughborough. I needed help and support. Then one day someone mentioned counselling. My initial thoughts were 'why do I need counselling?' I had thought about being a counsellor but needed to know more about it. So I found the courage to go and investigate what it was all about.

To my astonishment I loved it! I was talking to a complete stranger about everything, knowing I wasn't being judged. Everything from growing up, family, friends, school, college, being bullied, university, independent living came spilling out. You name it, I mentioned it! I felt empowered and free. I looked forward to going every week. I was beginning to find out who Kerry really was at 24 years old. I suddenly came out with: "I'm Kerry, I'm not trapped in a disabled body, I can achieve anything I want. I'm not going to hide in a spastic body any longer; I'm going to be counted for me. "I turned the word 'spastic' into a positive; Yes, I am a spastic, yes I can achieve. What is a name anyway? It is what I am. I was born a spastic; I will die a spastic. People know what a spastic is and I use this term in a positive way to educate and allow people to feel at ease with my abnormal body movements and speech.

After counselling I was more empowered and determined to achieve anything. I hadn't realised how the years of bullying had affected me and now I was coming to terms with my disability, which meant such a lot. No more letting people's attitudes grind me down.

Butterfly, Why can't I fly?

All around me butterflies are flying.
I can't why?
All the time I try,
But I fall to the ground.

I'm happy now,
But no one had the nerve to tell me why I couldn't fly.
For years, everyone has tried to make me fly.
I wanted to spread my wings and fly.
Just like the other butterflies,
But my wings wouldn't let me.

Doesn't matter now,
As I have learnt to grow,
By striving towards my goals.
All this, without being able to fly.

Not getting trapped in any webs,
Or tied down by people staring and saying, "Oh bless that poor butterfly."
But I know I'm a beautiful butterfly.

My Right Leg

My right leg
Spastic body
I need everything intact
Able minded
Spastic body
Wins all the time
Spastic body … used and abused
Been great for 30 years
But I push and push
Hoping to turn a spastic body
Into an able one……..
Does it work?
Spastic body loses to an able mind

A broken hip
Yippee such joys
Now what?
Pain…
Heartache…
Agony…
Misbelief…

Misdiagnosis…

Morphine…

Patronising…

A husband

My bloody spastic body!

My Accident

My life seemed all mapped out when I moved to Loughborough to a university town, back to where I belonged. Then came the crunch and my world felt like it was crumbling around me. I had moved to Loughborough to be with someone I thought would be my future husband, but it turned out not to be.

I really enjoyed my volunteering role and was benefitting as much as the children. I felt like I had a purpose. I felt frustrated and angry but also determined and happy. I knew I had to get my life back on track. I wanted to get back into a school environment to help disabled kids to learn and accept their disabilities at a young age instead of having the shock of their lives in their twenties. I wanted to give children with cerebral palsy the opportunity to talk about feelings around their disability and limitations.

One day after the school day had finished, a member of staff gave me a hand to get back in my car. I was busy chatting away to her, misjudged the pavement and fell out of my wheelchair. I felt so embarrassed. I jumped into my wheelchair, brushed myself down and got into the car without a fuss. I carried on with my normal routine at home trying to forget the pain, hoping it would go away. I woke up in pain during the night and took a spasm tablet, which didn't help at all! Next morning, I was determined the pain wasn't going to get the better of me and went to the gym as normal to practice my walking. However, to my shock, I couldn't bear weight to stand up, let alone walk. I was so scared and disappointed. The fall seemed so minor; surely, I shouldn't be in this much pain for this length of time? Or should I?

My doctor checked me over and prescribed spasm tablets. To be fair to him, I was in so much pain it was triggering spasms. The doctor must have thought I'd had a major spasm attack despite telling him about my fall. I carried on as normal, struggling in pain and after several trips to the doctor and a lot of diazepam and strong painkillers, I was beginning to think it was part of cerebral palsy. But, deep down, I knew I had to keep strong despite the lack of intervention from the doctors.

If I was able-bodied, they'd have sent me for an x-ray straight away. Eventually, I got to see a locum doctor who listened to my whole story. He was horrified to learn what had happened and that I was driving my wheelchair whilst on a morphine- based drug. I should have been in bed – at the very least. For the first time, a doctor was determined to get me the help I needed. I was placed on the waiting list for an appointment to see a neurologist. I was getting somewhere at last. Meanwhile I carried on with my life trying to survive as a single woman in my new hometown.

I got a placement at a local secondary school to teach on a social care course about disability. This helped take my mind off the constant pain. I enjoyed the placement immensely and I felt I broke down a lot of pre-conceived attitudes about cerebral palsy. Eventually an appointment came through for me to meet Mr Kershaw at The Nuffield private hospital under the NHS waiting list. I had mixed feelings about this appointment as I had spent the last six months trying to convince doctors and health professionals I had an injury rather than just bad spasm. I was pleasantly surprised to learn that Mr Kershaw was an expert in cerebral palsy and understood straightaway where I was coming from.

But because I was an NHS patient, I had to go back on their waiting list to receive treatment. So I got straight back into life, trying to forget about the appointment with Mr Kershaw and not get my hopes up too much waiting for a letter. I carried on applying for jobs as a mentor, trying to push the pain to the back of my mind like nothing had ever happened. Then, six weeks before Christmas, I heard the phone ring. This made me go into spasm and I fell onto my bad hip. Luckily, my friend Steve was due to visit me with his baby daughter and came to my rescue. He put me back to bed and sorted stuff out.

However, after a trip to the toilet, I fell again. I was trapped between the toilet bar and the toilet. We had little alternative but to call for an ambulance and I was rushed to the Leicester Royal Infirmary.

I was in so much pain and distress they placed me on a morphine drip and put me in traction. All this six weeks before Christmas! I really wanted and needed to return home as I had an interview the next day for a mentoring position. But after a lot of persuasion, morphine and traction, I was transferred to an orthopaedic ward full of old people, mostly waiting for hip replacements! I stayed there for six weeks.

Tom Cruise

Since the first time we met
I knew we were in for a challenge
My eyes gazed across the ward
I didn't know if I was high on pills
Or if you were Tom Cruise

All I knew was that I was at
An alone isolated point in my life
I'd just been through shit and back
My life had been turned upside down

High on morphine
Low on self-esteem
You were the one to set me free

Skallagrigg and Scallywag Love Always

Our love is strong,
our love was said to be strong,
our love will never break.

Our hearts entwined,
our hearts and mind are two of a kind,
our hearts will never break.

Downs and ups, been through so much,
surviving against the odds,
our love is pure,
our love is sure,
our love is here until we are here no more.

Our minds are one, our minds will not be done,
our minds will never break.

Our souls, each touch,
our souls can last,
our souls will never break.

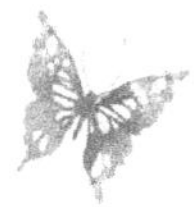

Meeting Chris

I can't believe I'm in this situation, I do get myself into some pickles but this one is actually unbelievable... I REALLY didn't want to be there. I pretended I was ok, but was at rock bottom again, high on morphine and spaced out. At least I was high, I suppose! I was on a ward with old people with broken hips and bones. A good time to be spaced out!

Eventually the morphine wore off and I met the other patients on the ward. I learnt very quickly I was the youngest. Most were old ladies and seemed a bit doolally! Opposite me was a really nice old lady called Maureen. We began to exchange smiles and, after a few days, started to talk. She was really lovely and kept my spirits up. I didn't have many visitors as I was new to the area and my family lived a fair distance away, so Maureen, or Mo as I called her, very kindly let me join in with her family visitors. It was lovely, it felt so natural. Over the next few weeks I met the whole family or so I thought. I had them all helping me at meal times and giving me drinks through a straw! I really hoped Mo didn't mind.

Then Mo had a visitor I hadn't met before. He looked similar to her other sons, but I wasn't sure. It could have been Tom Cruise, for all I knew, high on morphine! For some reason, when this guy walked through the ward, I got butterflies. I don't know why, maybe I needed a pee! He was able-bodied, stocky and quite fit! His smile took my breath away. Mo told me he was her youngest son Chris and he didn't visit often because he had no transport.

However, over the next few days and weeks, Chris started to appear more regularly and after a few visits we had a brief conversation. He asked me what I was listening to on the hospital radio and I replied, "Abba, Dancing Queen." It's my favourite and still is. We exchanged phone numbers. I was so pleased and excited! Deep down I was wondering how the hell I was going to text.

I hadn't even mentioned my cerebral palsy. What was I doing? What was I thinking? All I knew was I felt happy, excited and normal for the first time in years. I asked the nurses to help me with texting. I took the chicken's way out by loaning Chris a copy of Skallagrigg so he could get to know disability and how CP affected me. I thought this would be a good opportunity to teach him about my way of life whilst being laid up in a hospital bed. I couldn't believe it when Chris told me he had watched Skallagrigg for the tenth time in two days and knew it word for word! How amazing was that? But it meant so much to me.

A few days later Mr Kershaw wanted to talk about my hip and what he had found. Chris heard he was about to deliver the news and made a special effort to visit his Mum so he could hear what Mr Kershaw had to tell me.

That night he arranged for the nurses to wheel my bed into the visiting room so we could have a fish and chip supper and discuss the options Mr Kershaw had given me. It was magical. He made me feel so special listening to my worries about the operation.

The more I got to know Chris, the more time I wanted to spend with him. I felt like a teenager. One evening Chris arranged with the nurses for me to leave the ward for a few hours to get a change of scenery. It seemed like we were walking for ages down the long corridors of the hospital. Eventually we stopped in a deserted corridor and shared our first kiss. For me it was a dream come true; an able-bodied guy really interested in me and wanting to share my world! Chris wanted to find out everything about me and was willing to take my cerebral palsy on board. It was amazing, someone taking me for me and seeing beyond my disability. I didn't want my fairy tale to end and wake up from this dream. I was going through hell physically but at the same time meeting my Tom Cruise. How could this happen? It felt so natural.

Throughout my stay in hospital, I met the whole family including James, Chris' son. They were all lovely, helping me with food and drink whenever they could. James was a total credit to his parents, a very mature 14-year-old with a head on his shoulders. Weeks passed and our relationship blossomed.

Then it was crunch time as Mo was due to be discharged. I felt like I was losing part of my family and wondered if it would mean an end to our new relationship. My bubble was slightly bursting. I was selfish. I was going to miss Mo and didn't want to say goodbye to Chris. I knew I had to wake up from my dream at some point, I started to have feelings for this guy.

A few days passed and I was beginning to get back on track and survive without Mo, Chris and the rest of the family. The worst times of the day were fast approaching, visiting times and feeding! I looked around the room and all the other patients were sharing good times with their visitors and I was wondering what I was going to do for the next two hours and whom I could call to help me feed. I heard footsteps coming towards my bed. Butterflies crept into my tummy and a voice said to me: "Would you like me to help you feed?" it was Chris. He had walked eight miles to visit me! I couldn't believe my luck. I had tears in my eyes. I knew I wasn't dreaming and this guy was for real. I'd only just met him but already knew he was my soulmate, my equal. We spent the next two hours talking, laughing and getting to know each other more. Despite walking eight miles there, he had arranged a lift home!

Chris continued to see me in hospital. It was fantastic spending time with him and I knew this was going to last.

The day of my discharge was fast approaching and I dreaded having to say goodbye to Chris, as I knew the distance between our hometowns was going to present a challenge. I returned to my home in Loughborough and settled back into daily life just waiting for my operation date to come through. A few hours later I received a phone call from Chris asking if he could visit me. I was over the moon but scared, as I hadn't met him away from the hospital before. I didn't know what to do or think. He wanted to come over for a meal. I said I would pay if he would cook! He agreed. That evening we had steak, chips and asparagus all cooked with his very own hands. He left the washing up till the next morning though!

We had to face certain people's attitudes about our relationship, particularly as he was able-bodied and I'm a spastic. But the more opposition we got, the more determined we were to make it work. We wanted to enjoy our time together and show people we were meant to be. Through the early stages of our relationship, we had our fair share of challenges. Mo, bless her heart, passed away and this upset Chris immensely. I had to be his rock and support him through his darkest moments. It was tough but we came through, survived our experience together and it made us a strong couple. I managed to pick Chris up when he reached rock bottom. Now it was time for him to be my strength as I had my operation to contend with.

My operation was a huge hurdle for both of us. It was supposed to be simple and straightforward but turned out to be complicated with the recovery taking a lot longer than first thought. Chris was there every step of the way, wiping away my tears and laughing with me. We went through hell and back in the early days, but we were strong and remained positive for each other.

Chris is my soulmate, always has been, always will be. We see life through the happy and bad times and we know that we will always be there for each other, no matter what. So, in a way, I'm glad I fell out my wheelchair and broke my hip!

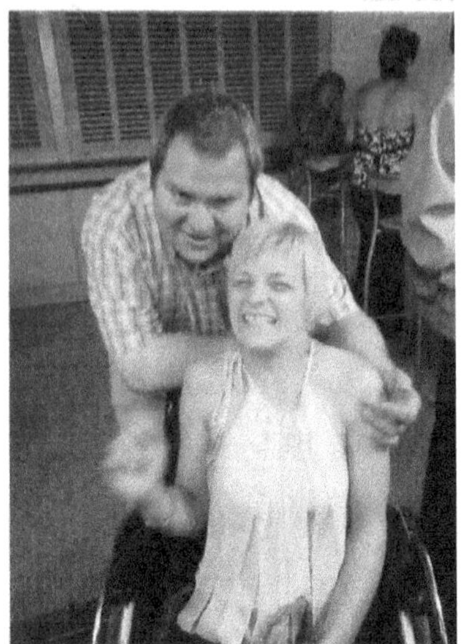

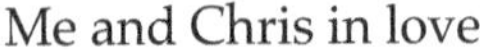

Me and Chris in love

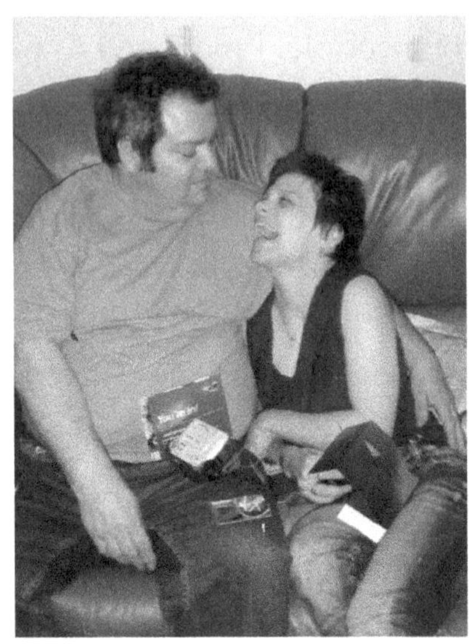

My soul mate

Creating Awareness

It's good to be different
It would be boring if we were all the same
I like being me
My own person
My own beliefs
My own values
My own challenges
I like being unique
Why be shoved in a box!
And labelled
I like being me
It's good to be unique
Let's celebrate difference
Let kids know it's good to be different
Let's create awareness and be different

I'm me and I love it

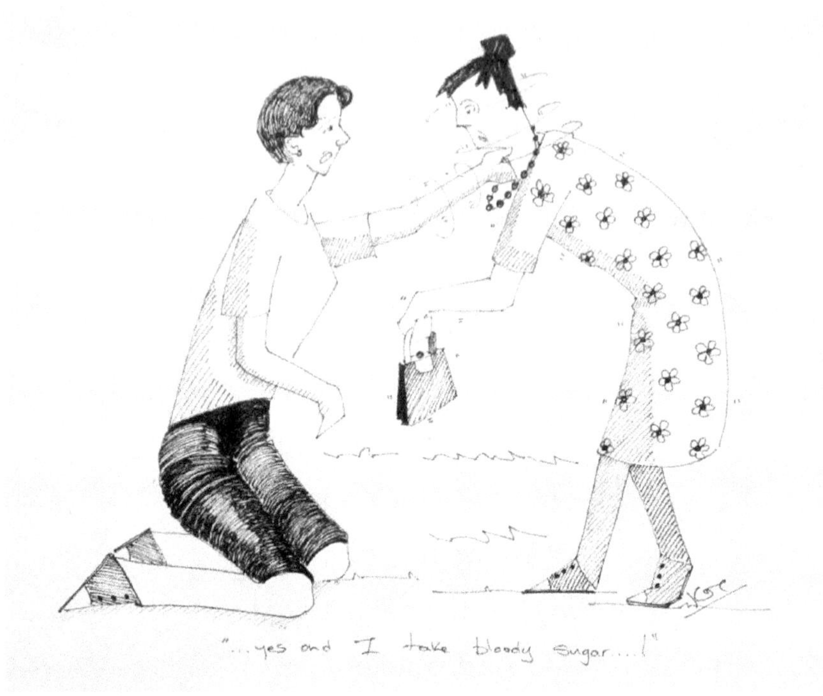

Illustration by Kevan Thompson to demonstrate people's patronising attitude towards disabled people

I really don't expect everything to come to me on a plate. You have to grab opportunities and make the most of what you can because sometimes they don't come to you.

Believe me, I don't live my life in a disabled way, I take every opportunity I'm given and rise to the challenge. It's the best and only way. You need to be strong in your outlook and determined to succeed. It's a big cruel world out there and you have to be counted like everyone else. I often say disability is like death. People don't know how to react when someone's just died and shy away from the situation, instead of confronting their fears and facing it. Death is so natural, an integral part of life. A bit like disability really. People don't know what to say to a disabled person, so they either don't say anything at all or the most stupid things.

Until this barrier is broken down, there will always be a gap between able-bodied and disabled. There is a big difference between adapting buildings for accessibility and altering often negative attitudes.

Children and young people are brilliant. They are not born with a preconceived attitude and tend to say it as it is, which I believe is the best policy. You can challenge and change children's ideas about disabled people, after all they are our next generation and once they know and understand about disability then barriers are ultimately broken down. Kids will say what adults want to say but can't, they just come out with it and it's all out in the open, I just feel this is the best way to educate; it's older people who are often stuck in their ways. This reflects the way society has viewed disability in the past.

In the year 2000, with the help of a really dear friend and colleague Jane Howard-White from Bedfordshire Scope, we received a Millennium Grant for cerebral palsy awareness and developed a tailor-made project to present in mainstream schools throughout Bedfordshire and Northamptonshire, ranging from reception to sixth form.

The project was based on personal experience as well as practical exercises for the young people to experience first-hand what cerebral palsy can be like to live with. For example, I got students picking up 5p pieces from the floor with oven gloves on, then watching me do it. Also writing their name using their opposite hand whilst watching me. I jumped out my wheelchair whilst the young people were sitting on the floor, so they had to confront their worst nightmare towards disability.

Another exercise was this: I picked on two volunteers as all the other students watched and concentrated on what I was going to do! I sat one child on a chair and told the other to stand behind it. I then deliberately talked solely to the child standing behind the chair, ignoring the child sitting down. In this activity it demonstrates to young people what it's like to be in a wheelchair and have someone talk over your head and totally ignore you, even when that person is talking. This can be one of the biggest barriers between able and disabled people, as some able-bodied people just presume that disabled people can't communicate and therefore just talk over their heads. I wanted to emphasise this quite strongly to young people as they are our next generation and if you educate them, they will know to direct questions at the disabled person. After two or three minutes I asked the others if what I was doing was right. I always received the right answer, thank God! That I need be talking to the child sitting down. I then explained that some young people and adults in wheelchairs can't verbally communicate. However, people should always direct the questions towards them and talk to them first and foremost as they know the right answer!

I usually finished the sessions with tailor-made poems and a question and answer session allowing the young people to ask whatever questions they wanted knowing they would receive an honest response. This was somewhat brave of me depending on the age and ability of the group! Questions ranged from 'Would I be able to walk?' to 'Would I be able to have a family?' Very thought provoking, interesting and mature questions. You could always see the teachers cringe at this part of the session. Hopefully I reassured both parties with my responses and only delivered age-appropriate answers. Talk about thinking on your toes! I certainly was using my brain during these days!

The millennium project sadly came to an end and it was time for me to move on and concentrate a bit more on my cerebral palsy as I had neglected myself for a long time. Time didn't stand still for long and soon it was time for a new challenge! I was approaching my late twenties and wanted to be like a student again (no study, just the drinking bit!). But, as always, this came with a challenge. Just going to local pubs and clubs was a bloody nightmare and hassle. I couldn't spontaneously ring up a friend and ask if they wanted to go for a drink. I always had to organise my pub route, making sure I could get in and out as well as use the toilets.

Pubs were generally quite accessible but, if I needed a pee, I had to think again! It was usually a cleaning cupboard that needed emptying to use! You couldn't swing a cat in them let alone if you needed help. Forget looking at yourself, as there was no mirror. No way of buying sanitary pads/Tampax or condoms either. So, if you are on a date, you're knackered!

Once at uni I wanted to go clubbing with friends. As always, I checked it out beforehand but, much to my horror, we were confronted with a rude arrogant shit of a bouncer who basically ignored me and talked directly to my friends saying I was a fire hazard and couldn't go in. However, we were determined to have a ball that night. After a lot of raving and ranting we entered that bloody club! We partied until the early hours, let our hair down, boogying in my wheelchair and not letting people's attitudes get in the way of a fun night. If people stared I just thought it was because people fancied me or wanted a snog! … maybe it was or maybe I was just pissed like everyone else! Whatever the reason we had a brilliant time, not letting people's reactions or attitudes spoil our night. To me that's what it is all about. Sitting on your arse moaning and complaining about stuff will get people's backs up. Get in there, be counted and prove you are just like anybody else. That's my way for challenging and changing attitudes.

Whenever I go shopping and someone stops and asks if they can help, I always say 'yes' whether I need it or not. This may sound weird but I feel that person has built up the confidence and courage to talk and confront a disabled person and that, if I knock them back, they may not bother to ask again. But when I need a box of Tampax it's just my bloody luck that the only passer-by is a young bloke!

Life is a challenge but it's what you make of it and how you rise to it. You need to be strong, determined and have a wicked sense of humour to survive but anything is possible, I am pleased to say. Buildings, public transport, attitudes and integration are slowly changing for the better.

Let's Go On Holiday

Let's get up and go
Let's spread our wings and fly
Let's go sailing
Let's go camping
Let's go all-inclusive
Let's be young
Let's be careless
Let's be responsible
Let's go on holiday!
We can, we can, we know we can

Or can we!?

After graduating from university, I decided I deserved a much- needed holiday. So a friend and I did some research and boarded a plane to Lanzarote. We had the best time ever. The accommodation was fab, in the form of studio apartments.

These were fully accessible and made our holiday complete. We did sunbathing, relaxing and drinking, just what the doctor ordered!

Several years went by and, after the breakup of my engagement, I wasn't going to miss out on a much-deserved holiday, so my old school teacher Leah and her husband Ian with their daughter Natalie stepped in and we all went on what should have been my honeymoon to Denmark. It was a honeymoon with a difference! We made the most of our week especially after losing two cases of clothes and having no change of underwear for two days! I couldn't believe waiting for our cases when everybody was whizzing round grabbing their cases. Finally, Ian grabbed his and I thought any minute now ours will come shooting down, but that minute seemed to last a lifetime as no more cases came down. Sheer panic hit mine and Leah's face and reality sunk in that there were no more cases on the conveyor belt. We had no clean knickers between us! Sheer panic entered! We were left without clean clothes for 2 days!

Another day we walked miles to see the famous statue of The Little Mermaid but were very disappointed when we finally got to see her. We had had to walk across woods and up hills with me and Natalie moaning our heads off and crying every so often, we really weren't amused with the situation. Again, I did my research into Copenhagen and the travel agent reassured me it was the best place for sightseeing for people in wheelchairs. However, when we arrived, the streets were all cobbled and most of the shops were located up steep steps. I had no chance of accessing the shops and the travel agent had said this was an accessible holiday. Accessible for whom? I suppose it's another tick off the list!

I really enjoyed spending time with my best friend and her family despite me and Natalie, Leah's daughter, being mournful for the loss of our relationships. I felt so sorry for Leah and Ian having to cope with heartbroken pre-menstrual youngsters.

Soon after meeting Chris, a year to the day that I split from my ex-fiancé, we decided we needed a holiday after all we had been through in a short period of time. After several conversations and research, it was decided we would go to Fuengirola in Spain. This was for two reasons. It was where Chris's mum used to go on holiday with her auntie and uncle and, secondly, Chris found it delightful I couldn't say where I was going! To his horror, I practiced like mad and became an expert at saying Fuengirola. Anyway, because we were new to booking disabled holidays, we left the capable job to my father as he had years of experience in this field. We had been on lots of family holidays over the years and he knew what to look for with regards to access and accommodation, or did he?

Chris and I were excited to be boarding a plane on our first holiday. We checked in with our luggage and were told to go to another department to check the wheelchair and batteries in before boarding. After a short flight to Fuengirola, we were helped off the plane and collected our luggage before boarding a taxi with a ramp. It was almost midnight when we reached our hotel, everything looked brilliant. There were ramps and lifts and in the hotel room everything was spot on, including bars in the bathroom and a walk-in shower. All seemed to be going without a hitch until next morning at breakfast we seemed to be waiting forever for a lift. The reason became clear when we entered the dining room. There were another 30 other people in wheelchairs but no other able-bodied people in sight. I felt so sorry for Chris!

We made the most of our holiday and loved the time we spent together. The hotel was completely wheelchair friendly, which wasn't a major problem, but still came as a major shock. After this holiday we decided to take matters in our own hands. I took sole responsibility for booking further holidays checking up access and accommodation. We spent many happy holidays together in places such as Cyprus and Spain.

We chose Las Vegas as our destination when we got married in 2009. Chris organised the whole affair. All I had to do was choose my dress and learn to stand on my own two feet again. It was absolutely brilliant having someone to take charge of everything. It was a bit like the TV reality show Don't Tell the Bride! Chris had visited Las Vegas a few years before and always wanted to return but never dreamt it would be to get married. It was absolutely fantastic. But I was quite shocked to discover how backward America was for disabled accommodation. I was quite disappointed with the standard of accessible accommodation.

As always, planning and organizing wasn't as straightforward as it should've been. I left the logistics to Chris but still had to think out of the box for long haul flights and going for a pee!

The loos on a plane hardly accommodate one person let alone two - add spasticity into the equation and Kerry and it could be a total disaster or an adventure. Perhaps I should wear a nappy instead?! Anyway, a few weeks before our departure, I gave the nappy wearing thing a trial run. Like most people, I hadn't worn nappies since I was a baby and was a little apprehensive to say the least but anything was worth a try.

First part of the experiment was to see how many wees the nappy would hold! I think three big wees was the record. Even after a week, I felt so unnatural weeing in them, I'd end up going in spasm with my muscles tensing so I gave up on the idea. After a lot of bubbly on the plane, I found myself having to use the loo in the first class cabin. The hostess was fantastic and cornered off the loo to enable Chris and I to have a wee.

Our wedding and honeymoon went without a hitch. We had ten nights in Las Vegas. After our wedding day we continued to explore Las Vegas, taking in some of the sights and scenery, and touring the strip. It was incredible! Everywhere was completely accessible and we were able to access all the strip facilities without any thought about disability access. The only problem we came across was the electric wheelchair that we hired ran out of juice! We had to stop frequently at different hotels for much needed alcohol beverage in order to charge the wheelchair. Staying at the place for an hour or two at a time!

We made the most of what Las Vegas has to offer, including winning on the blackjack tables!

And, after the wedding, we continued to enjoy holidays together.

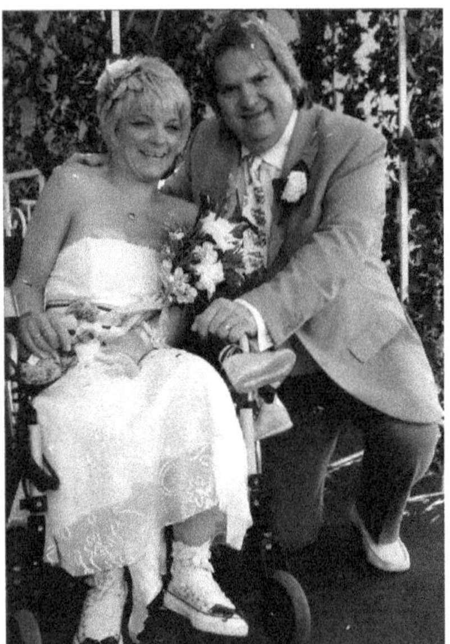

Las Vegas wedding!

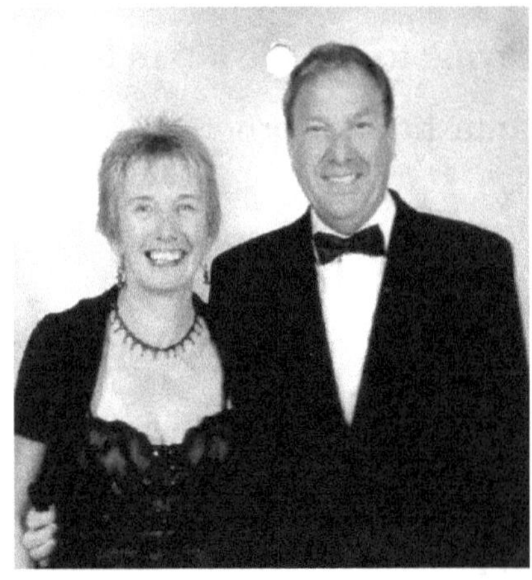

Leah and Ian

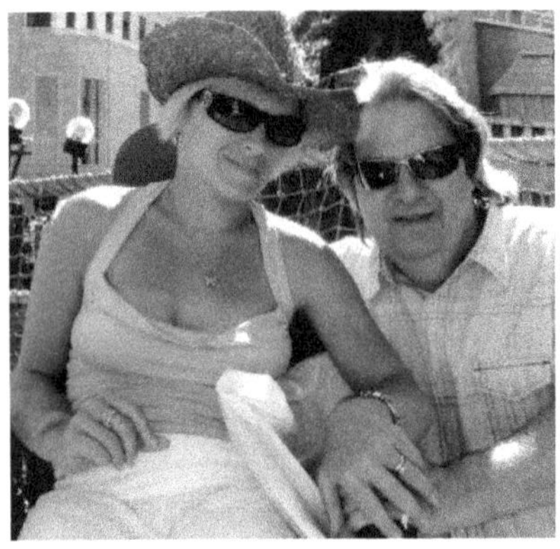

Honeymoon

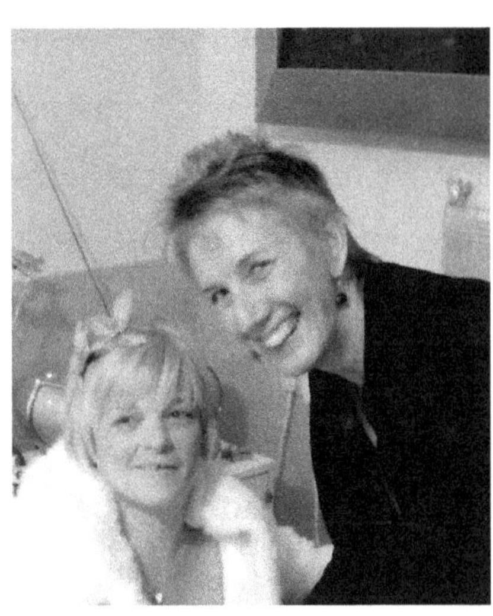

Me and Leah

Days To Remember

I'm Kerry
Boring old Kerry
Can't do anything
Won't do anything
I'm a spastic
Can't go places
Can't do things
I'm boring old Kerry

Oh, wait a minute
I just remembered
I have had an interview for Sky TV
And Pebble Mill at One
Been to The Savoy Hotel
Kicked Prince Charles
And had a garden party at Buckingham Palace
Met Tony Blair at Number 10 Downing Street
And asked Richard Wilson to pass a straw

So yes I am boring Kerry or am I!?

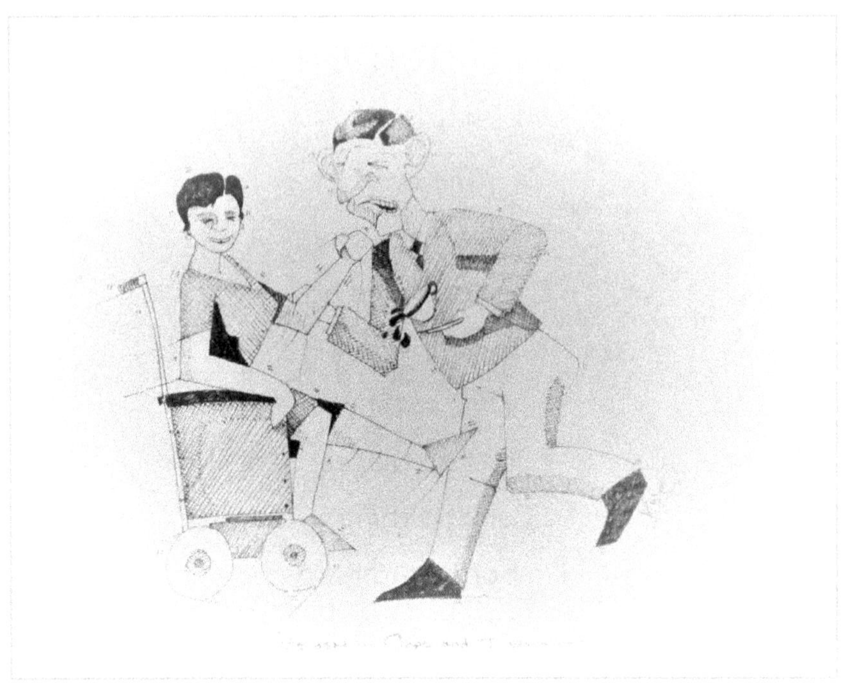

Illustration by Kevan Thompson, kicking Prince Charles!

I have met some incredible people and enjoyed some amazing experiences throughout my life. Here are some of the highlights!

It all began when I was 15 years old and got involved with The Prince's Trust. I was trying to get financial assistance for a mash garden we were creating at school, working alongside a local mainstream boys' school. This included writing to The Prince's Trust for funding. I not only received a grant for the project but was nominated for the Best of Britain Youth Award in 1988. I couldn't believe my luck. The competition was to celebrate and recognise the success of young people and there were 500 nominees, both able and disabled.

I was invited to the headquarters in London to have an interview. It was surreal; I couldn't believe it was happening to me. A few weeks later I was told I'd made the final 10 and invited to lunch at The Savoy Hotel in London, alongside stars such as Kid Jensen, Maureen Gray and EastEnders' Nick Cotton. The Duchess of Kent presented the awards and I was overwhelmed that I had gained fourth place in the competition. Totally incredible. Later that day I was invited to do a live interview on Sky TV with Frank Bough. My confidence rocketed. I felt so at ease and comfortable. It was an amazing opportunity.

Later that year I was invited to a Christmas Party hosted by Prince Charles in London. Of course, I jumped at the opportunity! I couldn't believe what was happening to a 16-year-old schoolgirl. I had just wanted to obtain financial assistance for a garden project and here I was being whisked away to posh events! I was among 500 young people, Prince Charles himself made a special appearance and seven young people were selected to have a brief conversation with him. I was fortunate enough to be one of them. I think the wheelchair helped!

I felt a nervous wreck, all kinds of emotions going through my head - what would I say? Would he understand me and how I speak? I didn't have time to draw breath before it was my turn for five minutes of fame. When Prince Charles came to me, my cerebral palsy got the better of me and I went into spasm and kicked him! Not a lot of people can say they kicked Prince Charles and got away with it. I felt embarrassed and ashamed and let down by my cerebral palsy but eventually managed to see the funny side of it.

My next claim to fame came just a few months after when, again through The Prince's trust, I was invited to meet the Prime Minister Tony Blair and his wife at 10 Downing Street. Once again, I was selected to have a brief conversation with the Prime Minister. I was humbled and honoured by being given such an amazing opportunity but, deep down, I thought 'why me?' I really didn't want to kick the Prime Minister as well as the future King of England! Reflecting back now, I wish I had kicked him, as he completely ignored me and directed all the conversation at my mother! I couldn't believe what I was witnessing for the Prime Minister not being able to relate to a disabled young woman. Cherie, his wife, on the other hand, witnessed what had happened and quickly stepped in to diffuse the situation and managed to win me over!

My next big adventure was again led by The Prince's Trust as I was invited to attend a garden party at Buckingham Palace. I felt privileged enough to ask Leah to accompany me. We had a totally amazing day from start to finish. I felt like The Queen!

We spent a very special day together in London, treating

ourselves like VIPs. We had a truly awesome day walking around the Palace grounds, eating cucumber sandwiches!

In 1995 Skalligrigg was nominated for Best Single Drama at the BAFTA awards, I was fortunate enough to attend. This was absolutely incredible, in my wildest dreams I could not believe what I was getting involved with! I was 22 years old and attending the BAFTA awards in London, mingling with people like Billy Connelly who hosted the awards. I actually bumped into John Travolta who turned around and said, "Hi I'm John!" and my reply was, "Hi I'm Kerry!"– simple as that! I wanted to appear calm and collected but inside I was bricking it! How the hell could this be happening to me? It was like a dream. Again, I should be so lucky to have bumped into Kylie Minogue! This was so surreal. Throughout the ceremony everyone was calm and collected when receiving the awards. The nominations for each award are known but the winners are announced on the actual night. Then the moment of truth, it came to our category for Best Single Drama… Skalligrigg was up against tough competition including Pat and Margaret, starring Julie Walters. When I heard who we were actually up against I just slumped back in my seat as there was no way on earth that we would come anywhere near Julie Walters. Then all of a sudden it was revealed that SKALLIGRIGG had WON! I just couldn't contain my emotion and spasm so I just screamed! I really didn't know what else to do! I could not contain myself! I felt eyes were looking at me but thought sod it! It was just a surreal moment that my naiveite of show business took the better of me! After the ceremony we moved on to the Grosvenor Hotel for a sit down meal and further celebrations. It was there when I received a chocolate BAFTA award for my contribution in the film. It was a phenomenal evening, something from my wildest dreams. I was fortunate to have my on-screen dad, Bernard Hill, with me throughout the evening. We laughed and partied till the early hours.

As you can see, my life hasn't been boring! I have had some amazing opportunities and managed to grab and hold on to them without spasm taking its toll! Who knows what the future holds in terms of stardom?!

Life is what you make of it at the end of the day. You have to grab every opportunity you can and make the most of your life.

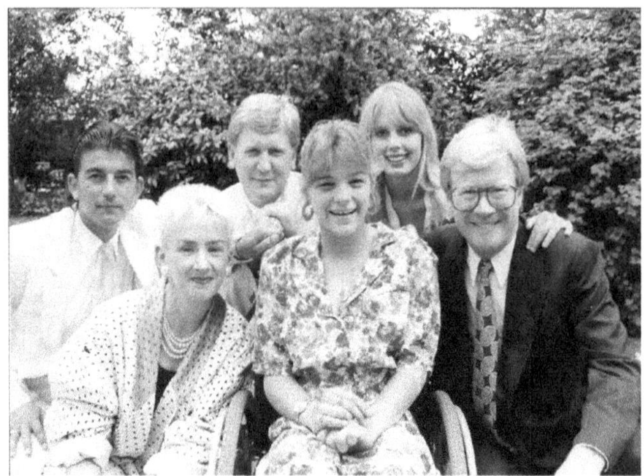

Me with all the famous celebs at the Savoy

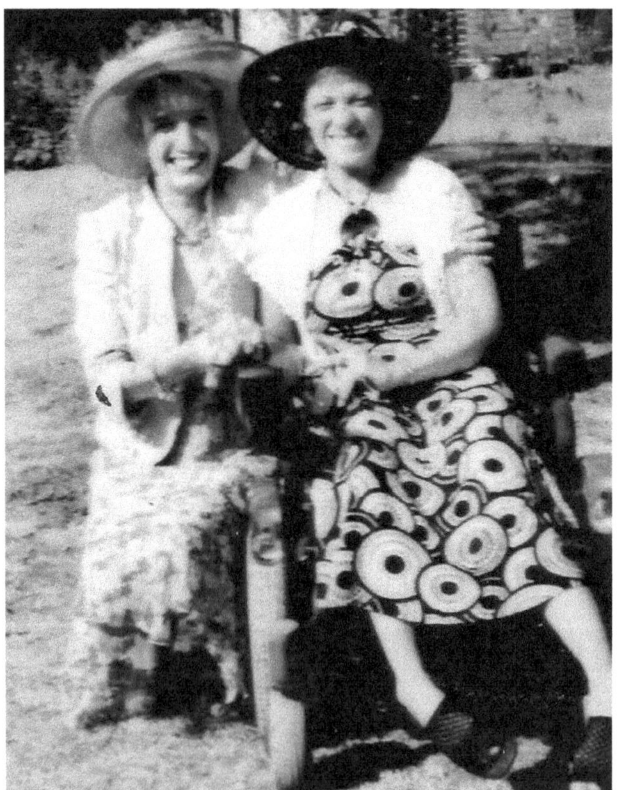

Leah and I before Buckingham Palace

Moving

It's time to go
It's time to get up
And lay our roots somewhere else
It's time to take that plunge
And go for it

It's time to spread our wings and fly
The family unit
Independent woman
A partnership
Back to the family unit
It's time to uproot
And spread our wings

Managing my own house
Every girl dreams of being in charge of her own destiny
School, college, then uni
Every girl dreams
Surely I can make it my dream too

I did! I achieved school, college and uni!

Now the biggest challenge ever
Independent living
Surely I can achieve this goal?

I may need help doing things but I'm in
Charge of my own destiny
It's been a challenge with its highs and lows

And faces that come and go
Starting out with 24-hour care
Was a nightmare that needed to be done
It shaped who I am today
Learning how to survive
Especially with an able mind but a spastic body
I survived
And learnt some great lessons on the way
I won't get trapped in any webs or tied down
Everyone has their own way of doing things
Just because I'm in a spastic body doesn't mean
I'm in a spastic mind
I'm in my right to make fuck ups
Take charge of my own destiny, like anybody
Or am I?

Moving house is a fundamental part of life but more interesting when you add disability into the equation!

On the whole it can be fun and exciting. When I was growing up, moving was a normal way of life as my parents were in the army. After the army, our first family home was a new build detached three-bedroom home in a cul-de-sac in the heart of Northamptonshire. It was a happy family home with minor adaptions. My parents had extra bars going up the stairs and bars fitted around the toilet. A downstairs extension was added to the property with a shower and toilet to be used by everyone. We stayed there for a number of years.

Our next family home was also located in Northamptonshire, a four-bedroom detached house with similar adaptions being made. Again it was decided to build an extension onto the property for greater independence as I was getting older and needed more privacy. So a shower room was built onto the downstairs toilet. This really made me feel brilliant.

After uni, like any other student, it was decided I wouldn't return to the family unit but would set up on my own. My name had been on the council waiting list for a property from the age of 16 and, after graduating in 1997, a ground floor property became available and I moved into my own home with 24-hour support.

The flat needed minor adaptions; it was wheelchair accessible and, once again, bars were fitted to aid my independence.

Minimal adaptions were made to the kitchen as I had live-in carers.

When I was 30 my life changed! I decided to uproot to Loughborough leaving my childhood years behind. After 18 months on the waiting list, I was offered a two-bedroom flat that was completely wheelchair accessible and just a short walk from the town centre. I grabbed this opportunity with both hands and spent many happy years there regaining my independence.

After many happy years and memories both Chris and I longed to create our own marital home and have a fresh start together. So we decided to apply for a house locally. We were placed on the housing list and had to wait for a suitable property. Once again it didn't take too much time for a semi-detached house to become available, 10 minutes walk from the town centre. Our first home together was brilliant. It already had a stairlift and so minor adaptions were needed to be sorted such as bars in the bathroom.

We have spent many happy years in our home but have come to the conclusion that I have come to the stage in my life now where my disability isn't working with me anymore, and once again it is time to uproot our home and look for a more suitable one. This maybe in the shape of a flat or bungalow, who knows what the future might hold?

Whatever the challenges will be, we will face them head on as the Coe team and we can do anything to achieve our goal.

Becoming A Mummy

What me…?
Pregnant Ahh
That blue line said it all
Yippee!
I'm going to be a mummy
Me a mummy?
Yeah that's right
Kerry a mummy!
A challenge
A life changing challenge
I can do this, I know I can.

Being a mummy
Oh wow!
Me a mummy
Oh wow!

Spastic mummy
Oh wow!
A mummy
Someone to look up to me

Someone who confides in me

Someone who loves me unconditionally

And I love them

A mummy

A spastic mummy

They see no difference

I'm Dylan-Grace, Charlie-Grace and Charlie-James'

mummy

It's wonderful

Two of them to take me for me

We get through

We're a team

James

In my hospital bed
There I lay
With my stepson ahead
There I met a vibrant young man
With years ahead

A spastic with so much to give
You took me in your stride
I took you in with pride!

Together we rise above
And the Coes will reunite

Charlie-Grace

Twinkle twinkle you are my star
Forever in my heart you are
Knowing you're there
And not so far

Charlie-Grace you are my girl
You came to us for a short while
Up above you look over us
You make us smile and that's enough

Charlie-Grace we love you so
In our hearts you're there to stay

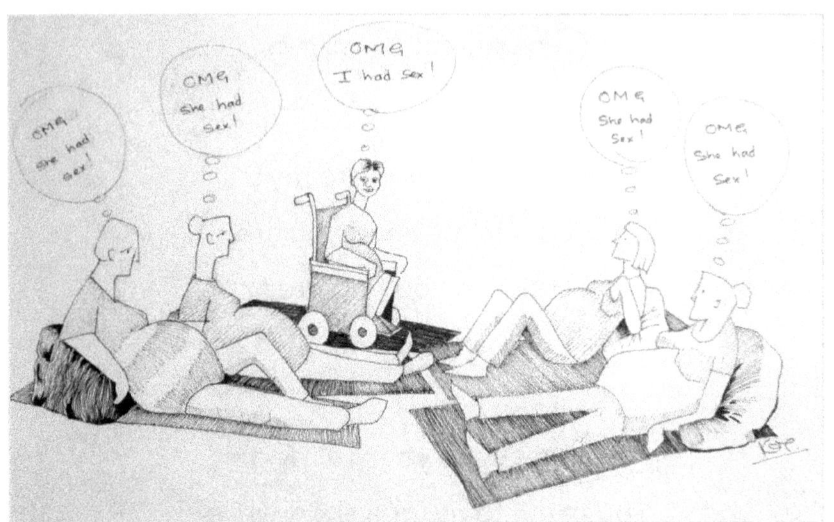

Illustration by Kevan Thompson, pregnancy exercise classes!

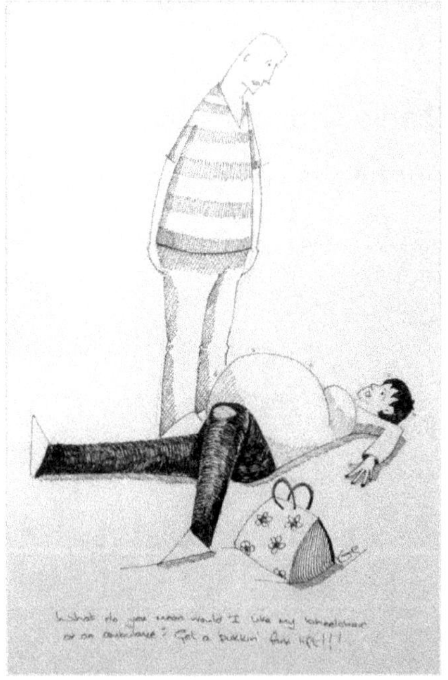

Enough is enough!

Just before Christmas 2010 I had a full day's training placement at Rainbows Hospice in Loughborough, where I was due to start after Christmas. I was really looking forward to volunteering for a charity who support sick and disabled children. Yet, after months of filling out application forms and receiving training, when the day actually came, I felt really off colour. It was weird. I didn't feel ill; I just felt strange with a funny taste in my mouth. I'd never felt like this before but was determined to make the most of the day.

I was excited about going out with Chris for a Christmas celebration with friends that night. Anyway, I muddled through the day feeling really crap. When I got home, I really wasn't in the right mood to go out but didn't want to let Chris and my friends down.

After doing my hair and make-up, I slipped a little black number on. My dress seemed much tighter than a few weeks before. I felt fat and frumpy and my boobs seemed enormous, but Chris reassured me I looked gorgeous. He would – he has always liked big boobs! I felt better about myself and was determined to enjoy the evening. But I didn't drink as I wasn't feeling right. Although we had a great night, my mood and body didn't pick up.

A few weeks later my period didn't come! We had planned to have a family after I came off all the medication. Our relationship was at the right stage to share our love and, after talking to James, my step-son, about his thoughts on being an older brother, we decided to go ahead. We enjoyed our practicing… and practice makes perfect! Never in our wildest dreams though did we think it would happen so quickly. It was like we were really fertile!

Anyway, when we bought the pregnancy test and did the necessary on the stick, we couldn't believe our eyes - the blue line was crystal clear. No doubt whatsoever, I was pregnant! I didn't know how I felt - happy, sad, nervous, excited, hormones everywhere. I suppose this was a normal reaction. I wanted to confirm my pregnancy so I booked an appointment with my doctor. I wanted to go on my own to get my head around the idea first. I didn't want Chris to be disappointed if the pregnancy test was faulty.

I received mixed reactions from the doctor, who wasn't my usual GP. I felt she judged my disability first and foremost as she confirmed my pregnancy. After a minute of silence, shock and horror, I felt excitement, happiness, contentment and fear! I burst out crying. I don't think the female GP knew what to do with such a reaction… After reassuring her I was overjoyed and happy, we talked about booking in for a scan. I decided which hospital to go to and made the appointment for the following week. When I told Chris the news, we were both on cloud nine and couldn't believe what was happening.

It was surreal but we both had fears to contend with. For me, it was about being a disabled mum and how I'd cope emotionally. I have always believed that a child should never be a carer for their disabled mum. I wanted to get my head around my care needs alongside my kids to ensure that wasn't going to be the case. Chris had other issues to deal with including being an older dad and taking the lead role in the physical care for the baby.

Once the shock was over, we were both overjoyed at the thought of becoming parents. We wanted to share our news but needed to wait for our first scan. Excitement got the better of us and James seemed the right person to tell. He was overjoyed and shared our happiness. I was so pleased we had his approval. It meant the world to me.

We set out on our new adventure the following week at the maternity unit. We felt scared surrounded by pregnant women wandering around with their pregnancy folders. They gave me mixed reactions. Perhaps they thought I was in the wrong department! Who knows? That all changed when I received my pregnancy folder. I was proud and excited as though I'd just been made a member of an exclusive society. I could almost hear people whispering 'she's had sex and she's disabled'. It was an amazing feeling of empowerment.

After several consultations and tests, I eventually met a lovely consultant, Dr Singhal, who was going to be with me every step of the way. She was willing to answer any questions I had. She had limited experience of disability in pregnancy, but knew everything else and in return I was the expert on my own body and so we worked together. Now we could work together throughout the pregnancy. She recommended regular scans just to make sure everything was running smoothly. I had no objections as I could see my bump grow and follow the heart beat all the way to the delivery suite. From the start, it was agreed that I would have an elective caesarean. This was mainly due to complications from my own birth and to reduce stress to the baby, especially if I was in spasm. I began to relax as I was in the best capable hands.

I enjoyed my pregnancy. I blossomed and my spasms actually went away, it was a miracle! I found this quite scary as my body movements were changing. It was good but my body took some getting used to it. I craved Bran Flakes and apples. Very healthy! I liked to talk to my little developing bump. I wasn't satisfied talking to a nameless bump so decided to give my bump a unisex name; Chris really liked the singer Bob Dylan and the alcoholic Welsh poet Dylan Thomas. So Dylan was our name for the bump soon to become our child. I sang, talked and played music. It was amazing watching our baby grow by having regular scans before finally at 20 weeks we were able to name her Dylan-Grace, as I loved the name Grace. I was so excited knowing I was having a little girl, a little me. Was the world ready?!

A friend mentioned a local private clinic doing 3D baby scans. I was so excited I booked straightaway regardless of the expense! The 3D scan was unbelievable, well worth every penny. It allowed us to bond further with Dylan-Grace, watching her move in my tummy brought tears of joy to my eyes. I continued to blossom throughout the pregnancy. I still had reservations about being a disabled mum, as I needed to know I could look after my baby and do as much as I possibly could for her. I needed to think outside the box and work out how I could achieve my aim, making sure people knew she was my daughter. I knew my limitations, or did I? After a long chat to Leah and a few friends, I signed up for a breastfeeding course as this would give me the sole responsibility for feeding my daughter. I could also challenge people's attitudes by physically showing that Dylan was my daughter. I didn't know if I could achieve this goal but was determined to give it a bloody good go! After the course, I continued to watch the DVD day in and day out. I think Dylan and I got bored.

My next challenge was to think about my care needs and working with my daughter. I wanted my daughter to see me as a strong independent mummy and needed support workers to understand how to facilitate my role as a mum without taking over. I needed the right people for the post who appreciated my outlook. This challenge was new for all of us. Support workers had to appreciate the level of support needed and when to step back. We certainly have learnt together and my team has stuck by me through thick and thin.

What about going out on my own? I needed to show the outside world I was mum, and my daughter belonged to me! I knew a charity that adapted equipment for disabled people and, to my amazement, they were willing to adapt my wheelchair to carry a car seat out in front of me. This again enhanced my independence. When the charity came up to visit and assess my needs, I couldn't believe the design that they had come up with. The car seat would be attached to a metal frame which in turn would be attached to the wheelchair and would swing in and out when needed. So me being me! It was great to be organised and thinking ahead of how to work through everyday practical challenges.

My Mummy

My Mummy is disabled
My Mummy is strong
My Mummy loves me
My Mummy is a hero
Because she cares for me

My Mummy is always right
My Mummy is the same
As any other Mummy
Except she is in a wheelchair

Dylan-Grace April 2017

Towards the third trimester of my pregnancy, I was beginning to be scared and concerned but I suppose every mum feels the same. I knew Dylan-Grace was really comfortable, as I had no signs of her coming out! It was a hot August day as my due day approached. My boobs were full of milk, my arse was aching, but I was so glad my C-section was the next day! It was arranged that Chris would be there throughout my hospital stay to help with my care needs and our daughter. We woke up really early with feelings of excitement, joy and worry. We didn't know what to say to each other, but we knew what to do - prepare for theatre. This was a challenge in itself. The epidural presented a lot more of a challenge than we first thought. How do you get a heavily pregnant woman to keep still on her side? Then add cerebral palsy!

The anaesthetist had several attempts to site the epidural and was about to give up when Dr Singhal stepped in. She talked to me to help me calm down and helped me stay still allowing the anaesthetist to get to work. Two minutes later we were ready for action. The C section itself seemed like I was on The Titanic, a weird feeling.

Twenty minutes later Chris and I heard the sound we had been waiting for - our baby daughter, Dylan-Grace, entering the world weighing 6lb and 13 oz through tears of joy. 'To begin at the beginning' were the words that came to Dylan-Grace's ears and our lives felt complete. It was truly amazing.

Whilst Mummy got sorted, Daddy and baby bonded. Time to put all our hard work to the test. Dylan-Grace instantly latched on to my boob; all our hard work preparing paid off. It was an amazing feeling. We got into a routine straightaway. Daddy got the shitty end and I got the boob end! Dylan-Grace stayed on my boob for 17 months. I was so proud of her, knowing exactly what to do, working with her Mummy throughout the spasms.

The best thing was not to be scared and just get on with it. But I was really scared leaving hospital and returning home, especially when Chris had to go back to work. I was really frightened about picking her up. I didn't want to go into spasm and drop her.

I remembered what a midwife had told me a few weeks before - she was my baby and had grown in my tummy; she wasn't a china doll and I couldn't break her. This was the best advice anyone had given me. I never looked back but just got on with it. Me and Dylan worked together as a team managing to join local mum and tot groups and just being a normal mum and daughter.

The wheelchair adaption was surely amazing and gave people a starting point for conversation. Whenever people judged me or wasn't sure if Dilly was my child, I would get her to feed on my boob. That soon gave them the answer! The adaption meant that Dylan was no more than 2 feet from me when we were both in the wheelchair. I could smell her nappy and she could smell her milk! This was a great advantage when people stopped and stared as I could just shove Dylan on my boob to feed and show people that she was my daughter. I always dressed Dilly in pink so it was blatantly obvious that she was a girl. However, I once had someone who clearly wanted to speak to me, come up and she obviously didn't know what to say so she asked if the baby was a boy or girl! Bless her, she must have felt so embarrassed afterwards. Other times when people were obviously working out what relationship we had as it is quite a taboo thing to see a disabled mum with an adaption on a wheelchair, carrying her own child. When this happened I often got Dilly to feed! So there was no shadow of a doubt that she was my daughter! When Dylan came along, we always knew as older parents that she would not be an only child. We wanted her to grow up with a sibling close to her own age. We knew James would protect and cherish her but equally felt she deserved to be part of a family and have a brother or sister to play with.

When Dylan was 4 months old I fell pregnant again. We were overjoyed and excited that Dylan Grace would have a brother or sister to play and grow up with. As older parents we really wanted Dylan to grow up with a sibling of a similar age, therefore I was delighted to discover that I was pregnant.

However, this was short lived. At just 10 weeks, I experienced back pains and bleeding excessively on the toilet. I knew that sadly I lost my baby. Sadly, everyone was trying to convince me otherwise but a mum's gut instinct knew. As it was Easter weekend, we had to wait a whole week for an emergency scan which confirmed my suspicions that I had miscarried. I knew deep down inside that I lost my baby the day I was bleeding on the toilet but Chris was still holding onto the doctor's words. I was determined to always remember our loss and for our family to talk openly about Charlie-Grace as death is a natural and integral part of life. I think it's important not to be scared of something so natural. We always celebrate Charlie-Grace's birthday and talk openly about her.

In line with advice following my miscarriage with Charlie-Grace, we waited a couple of months before trying to conceive again. Three months later, we were so delighted when I missed a period and discovered I was pregnant. Delighted and worried.

There were mixed emotions after the miscarriage. We decided to keep the pregnancy to ourselves. We had to wait for 12 weeks!

Once again, I was referred to Dr Singhal and my pregnancy seemed to go quite smoothly, losing my spasms and jerking movements again. It was harder this time as, having Dylan-Grace to care for, I was just like a normal mummy. However, when I was 24 weeks, I started to lose blood. I had an emergency scan and to our delight everything was fine and I continued with the pregnancy. We went for another 3D scan so we could see our baby son Charlie-James grow. It was amazing! No two pregnancies are the same. I was in and out of hospital with various issues. One of the main problems was sicking up blood! This suddenly happened every morning at 6am when I was 30 weeks pregnant. It was so scary and worrying but, as I was in hospital at the time, Dr Singhal arranged a cat scan to investigate why. It was very risky but sicking up blood presented its own risks. After a lot of consideration I decided to go ahead with the scan as if I didn't it could have presented more problems further down the line.

However, much to my delight, the results came back clear and within time it settled down.

A Mummy

Me a mummy
I love the way we work together as a team
Facing each new day head on
Don't care about people stopping and staring
We don't care
It makes us feel proud
No one can ever stop The love between us

A mummy, yes a mummy
Kerry-Jane Coe, a mummy

Mummy

I love mummy

Because she's my best Mummy
Ever!

Charlie-James, April 2017

During the third trimester, I was having a lot more spasms, which seemed like contractions. It was decided I would receive my Botox injections to help with the pain. I understood the risks and complications of having Botox in pregnancy, but this outweighed the pain and discomfort for me and Charlie-James. I also knew I couldn't have Botox for eight months after giving birth if I wanted to breast feed, which of course I did!

The injections were a huge success and I was able once again to lead a painless lifestyle. However, Charlie being Charlie, I was back in hospital at 37 weeks as I couldn't sit up in my wheelchair because of contractions / spasms. I wasn't too sure what it was as I had never experienced these feelings before. It didn't feel like a spasm, but I wasn't 100 per cent sure it was a contraction either as I had never experienced contractions with Dylan. I just knew it was strange and different.

Whilst I was at the hospital, consultants spoke about bringing my C-section forward two weeks. I wasn't happy or convinced it was the right decision as I always remember Dr Singhal saying try and carry as close to the due date as possible as this allows the baby to continue to grow with less chance of complications. I wanted to stick it out for Charlie-James. The consultant gave me a steroid injection before allowing me to return home before the C-section so I could see my daughter. This injection really hurt and I sobbed. When I got home I discovered my stairlift wasn't working. It was a Friday night and I couldn't get the engineer out till the next day, so I decided to sleep downstairs. This presented its own challenges!

Next morning Chris managed to carry me upstairs so I could have a bath and relax. Later that day my close friend Karen called round. She was absolutely brilliant, really supportive of me as a disabled mum. I was going to the toilet a lot and having a discharge but thought nothing of it. I was really tired so we went to bed early. However, I woke Chris up at 4am with severe back pain and wanting to go in the bath. I went back to bed after a long soak. Half an hour later I felt something cold and wet between my legs. I didn't know what the hell to do. It was a Bank Holiday Monday and Charlie-James wasn't due for another two weeks. Chris, being Chris, wanted to go back to sleep. I got him to ring the maternity unit for advice and they told him it sounded like I was in labour but not to panic – "Come in when you're ready but no need to break any speed records." Chris went back to sleep!

I got up needing the toilet. I was in agony and had feelings of wanting to push. Five minutes later I woke Chris who didn't know what to do. We rang Simone and Karen, who both dashed over as soon as they could. Karen asked Chris to call an ambulance which came within a couple of minutes. Simone and Karen managed the whole situation and Chris, beginning to panic, took charge of Dylan-Grace. Simone tried to work out how to get me from the bathroom to the ambulance! The paramedics confirmed I was in labour and gave me gas and air. It was a real challenge getting me downstairs, but we did it.

Then it was time to get on a stretcher and into the ambulance. The paramedics were amazing. I don't think they had ever met a spastic before, let alone one ready to give birth! They took hold of the situation. On the way to the hospital my waters broke… I was trying so hard not to fall off the stretcher in spasm as we turned a corner in a speeding ambulance! But this was so difficult as Charlie-James was on his way. We got to the delivery ward to be confronted by another challenge. How could I get from the stretcher to the delivery bed?

Without any hesitation, the paramedics lifted me…

As it was bank holiday, the midwives on shift didn't know me or my disability and weren't sure how I was going to deliver the baby! They must have wondered how I'd conceived in the first place! My body was all over the place. It felt like I had to teach them whilst trying to push a baby out! I decided the only way of getting Charlie-James out was to deliver on my side with someone holding my leg up in the air! Once in this position, it only took two pushes for Charlie-James to be born… It was incredible, amazing. I think Botox and a few spasms on the way helped Charlie to enter the world… I received a few stiches which again presented a challenge as I had to be stitched lying on my side!

After all the necessities were done, I was able to cuddle my son while he fed beautifully on my boob. It was an amazing feeling once again to be able to achieve breast-feeding for Charlie.

Chris soon entered the delivery suite and witnessed a beautiful sight of mother and baby bonding. He burst into tears and soon joined in the happiness. I stayed in hospital with Charlie for a few days to recover after the stitches and check everything was ok with Charlie. Then we returned home and settled into family life quite quickly. Dylan loved her baby brother to bits and the bond was inseparable from the start and has gone from strength to strength.

Life has moved on and we have adapted to living as a family unit. One of the traditions that I feel is extremely important is family holidays. These are cherished memories and valuable experiences. When Dilly was a baby, we took her on her first holiday to a Haven holiday park. We checked the accommodation was suitable not only for a wheelchair but a family unit. This was a double whammy as I had to be so much more organised and double check the accommodation for wheelchair and family suitability.

I often find that how companies interpret disability and adaptions are not universal throughout the hotel chains. This makes it incredibly frustrating when you are a family of four and the family room is not located next to the disabled room. I dread arriving at different locations to see what we are faced with.

You should look forward to a holiday taking in the sights and scenery without stressing over the suitability of the disabled hotel rooms.

For Chris' 50th birthday, I decided to surprise him with a trip to Lanzarote. Knowing I had already been to a suitable location and property, I decided to return to the same destination. It was fantastic. I secretly opened up a bank account without Chris knowing and even arranged his week off work. It felt really devious as I saved like mad for six months to make this happen for my loving, devoted husband. After not having much input for our wedding, this made me feel better about it. Four months into the surprise preparation, I discovered I was pregnant with CJ. I would be 34 weeks pregnant and not able to make the most of the all-Inclusive. I had to leave this in Chris' capable hands! I only told Chris two weeks beforehand that we were jetting off. We had a fantastic time with our daughter and our son in my tummy.

The four of us enjoy family holidays now. It is important to spend time together and lead a normal family life. It's a big challenge trying to tick all the right boxes, as you can't just pick up a brochure and decide where to go. You need to be well organised and well prepared. Anything is possible if you put your mind to it and think outside the box.

I would have never had my own family if I didn't think I could achieve my goals. Everyone has a different way of running and organising their family life and that includes us. Our children have grown up knowing Mummy needs a little bit more help and support, and I think it makes them stronger individuals. It equips them for life. I admit I'm too soft with them about tidying their rooms. I think it's because I can't do it myself. But I know they can do it if they need to! When on my own with them they help a lot more than is expected at their age. This has helped them grow up with a more mature outlook. They have certainly had a taste of disability and people's attitudes, which has equipped them for life on the outside world. They both know Mummy can't run to their rescue in times of need which makes them more independent and strong minded. Like Mummy, they don't let anything stand in their way!

I was determined from an early age to join local clubs and activities with them to enable them to mix with other babies and children. This gave them the freedom and space to explore their surroundings and be like 'normal' children. As a disabled Mummy, I was faced with positive and negative attitudes from groups and clubs alike. But yet again I was determined to show professionals and other mums that a disabled parent could achieve just the same as them.

Throughout my children's lives, I am honoured to make friendships with amazing parents, who allow their children to experience the world of disability without being scared. Both Dilly and Charlie are actively involved in community activities outside school such as swimming, drama, Brownies and beavers as well as several school activities at St Mary's Loughborough. Dylan has learnt how to sew so hopefully she won't be kicked out of Brownies like her mum! I don't want them to miss out because their mummy is disabled. I sometimes have to be creative and think outside the box, but I always manage to work through the challenges. The staff at St Mary's primary school have been really supportive to us as a family, offering help without any hesitation when I've needed additional support to carry out my role as Mum.

I'm a volunteer reader at school which enables pupils to come into contact with a disabled person. It is important for both my children and their school friends at such a young age as it allows them to mix with someone with a disability. This also enables me to offer Cerebral Palsy awareness within the school.

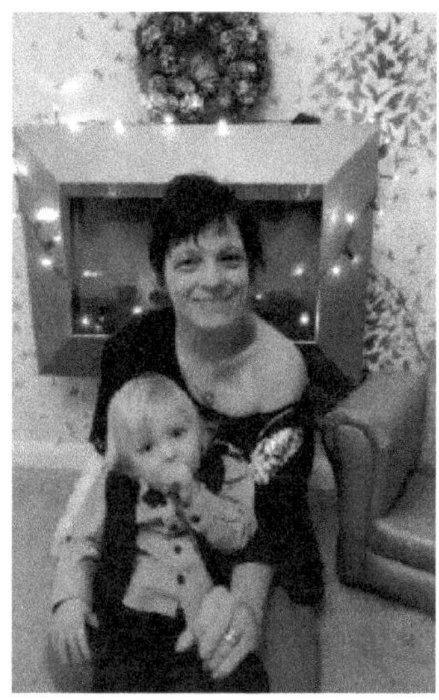
Me and CJ, 2015

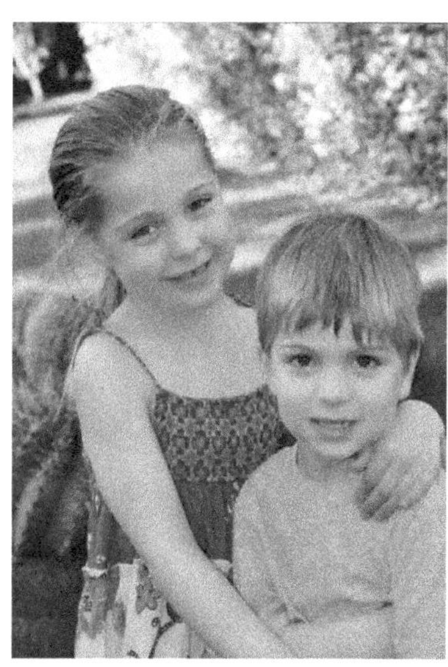
Dylan and Charlie

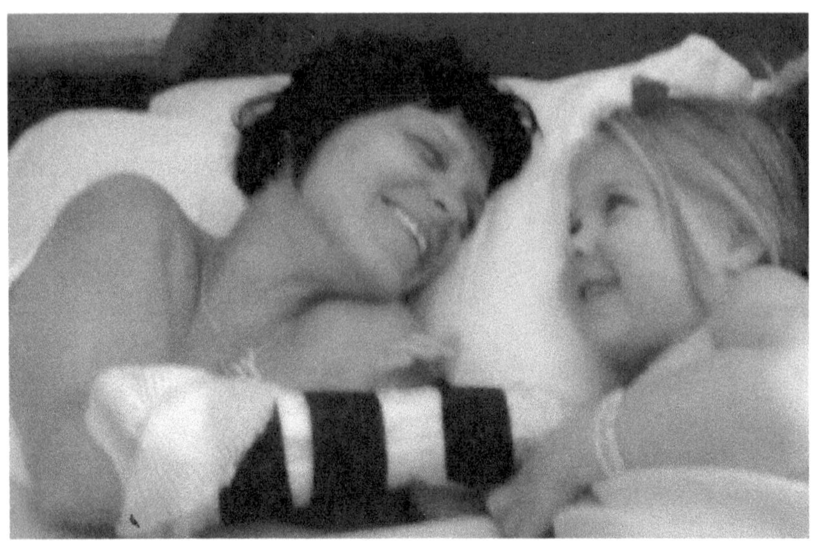

Me and my little girl

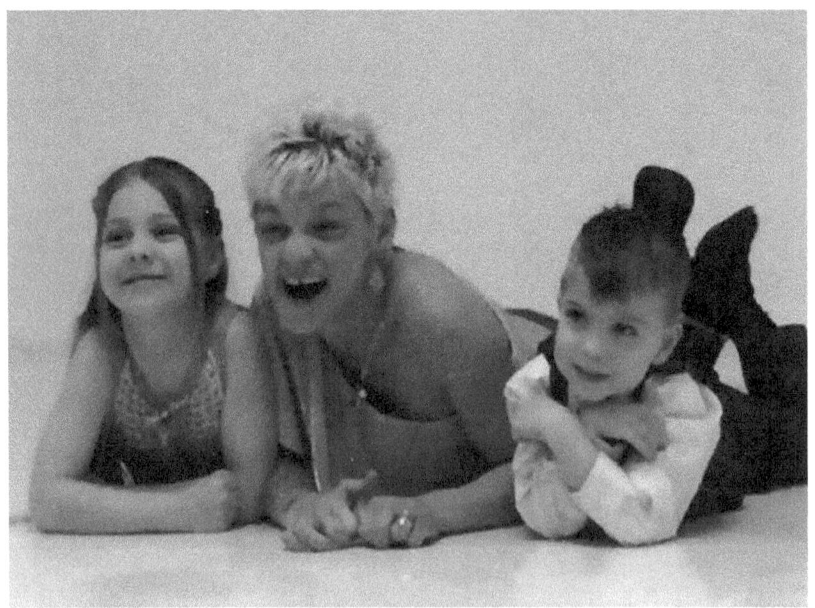

Me and my babies

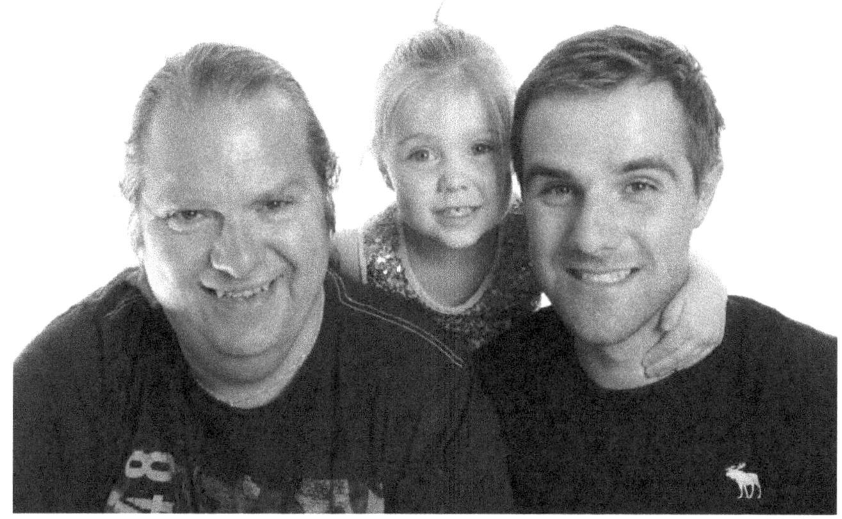

Chris, James and Dilly

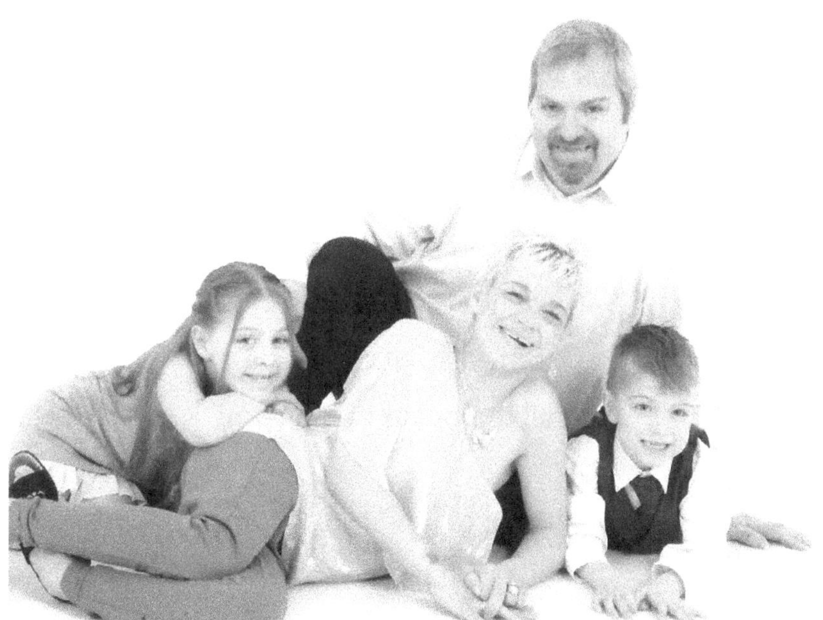

The Coe family

Growing Old

Old age
What joys
What thrills
Tears and laughter
Piles and wrinkles
False teeth
False hips
Grey hair
Saggy tits
What a state to get in!

It comes to everyone
But I'm used to a wheelchair!
I just need the wrinkles
But will that come
With all the Botox in my bum!

I just can't believe I am 45 years old and I'm writing about old age and how it affects me! I feel knackered just thinking about it... Some professionals claim old age creeps in earlier with cerebral palsy.

I'm bloody knackered already… Knackered body, good brain! The amount of Botox I've had over the last 15 years has helped me keep healthy and young for my age I think!! I admit I colour my hair to hide the grey, but doesn't everybody? On the whole I feel quite fit and healthy. My CP lets me down occasionally, but I pop the odd pill and keep up the Botox and that sorts me out… I don't like to rely on medication heavily especially for my CP as the dose will only increase over time and I'd become more docile! I was born with CP and I'll die with it… My CP comes with me, I don't go with it... So I refuse to take medication on the grounds of being a spastic but that's just me and my outlook.

My eyesight is shit and I need reading glasses but that goes with approaching your 50s… My hearing is crap but that's linked to my CP - I just cope with it. I do have selective hearing when it comes to Chris and the kids! But doesn't everyone…?! On a serious note, one thing that does cross my mind quite a lot is dentures! I worry about losing my teeth and how the hell they would fit dentures… Picture it, I'd be talking and the false teeth would be going the other way! And the amount of saliva I produce they wouldn't bloody stay in anyhow! I suppose the advantage is I could take them out to clean and know I'd cleaned my teeth properly without causing any damage!

Joking apart, one thing that often gets to me is when I go somewhere with a problem and the initial response is 'Do you think it's connected to your CP?' My gut reaction is I've never been here before, so you tell me if it's normal for my age group? Then we can rule out the CP part. There's nowhere to turn to about CP and old age because CP is as individual as individuals themselves. You never get two people with the same diagnosis. I love being so unique in some ways but sometimes wish I wasn't as unique and people could tell me what was wrong with my body: is it old age or is it CP?

I have pushed my body to extreme limits over the years but, if I had my chance again, I wouldn't change how I've lived my life. I just wish someone could tell me the difference between CP and old age. Growing old doesn't bother me in the slightest as it's a natural thing and everyone grows old. Sometimes it frustrates me that I can't get up and go. My brain is telling me one thing, my body another. I tend to listen to my brain over my body…

I want to be as independent as I can for as long as I can, this is a motto I have followed in my life. First and foremost, I'm a mum and my family come before my CP. Might sound like I'm in denial but believe me I'm not. I've learnt to cope and survive with CP and it's my way of dealing with it. I have fully accepted being unique and different and my body has fully accepted that it's got to come with me!

I've got the wheelchair; I just need the wrinkles!

I Am Able

Want to be able
Want to be strong
Want to be determined
Want to be me
I can do things
And be counted for me
It is hard to be able in a spastic body
But there's no turning back
As this is what I wanted all my life
This is ME

I would never have thought I'd be writing my story for others to be inspired and feel supported. I'm so glad to help individuals to live with cerebral palsy rather than cerebral palsy living with them.

As you can gather, I never let life get me down. I always find a way of achieving my ultimate aim - sometimes this can be quite easy, whereas other times can be a challenge. On the whole it's been fun and exciting. Life is what you make it at the end of the day. Now there is nothing that can get in my way! I see life as one big challenge and people are equal. Life can be shit sometimes, trying to juggle everything as well as cerebral palsy. I have a wonderful, fantastic husband who stands by me and supports me in all ways in everything I do. We learn together about cerebral palsy and old age. Who knows what's round the corner?

No one can tell me what to expect. I try not to think too much about it and concentrate on what I can do today. It's really hard and frustrating at times as I have already lost the majority of my physical independence. That's difficult as I have spent many years trying to get around my CP. I will just have to stretch those ways and learn different ones to achieve my aim but within a more spastic body than normal!

It is hard, sometimes impossible, but if I hadn't pushed myself all these years, I wouldn't have achieved my aims and aspirations. I no longer drive a car due to my hip and hand injuries. I do miss driving, especially having two young children, but at least I can say I've done it and ticked it off my list!

Today I live within my family unit - me, Chris and our two lovely children – with the help of my support package. I receive support from dedicated team members who support my needs both physically and my role as Mum. They are my hands, but not my brain! They understand the importance of me being independent. I still want to be able to "fuck up" and be in charge of my own destiny. Make my own choices, right or wrong, for both me and my family.

I continue to have Botox in my lower limbs especially during winter. I tend to have the injections every six months to keep me supple and as pain free as possible. I live my life in spasm and I don't know what it is to live without spasms, but Botox certainly helps me to live an able and pain free life.

I will never let CP stop me, never have done, never will… If someone says I can't do it, that makes me more determined to work through the challenge and survive in an able-bodied world. Sometimes this has come at a huge cost and I have put my body at risk but I wouldn't change a thing. I've already told you what happened in 2006 when I fell out of my wheelchair and doctors constantly put my hip pain down to CP. Similarly, in 2014, I was crawling in a group when I fell and twisted my wrist awkwardly. Deja vu came into play with doctors telling me it was all part of CP and I was in spasm when I'd injured my wrist…

I continued to live in severe pain, not allowing the injury to stand in my way. However, after 13 weeks and much perseverance, I discovered my wrist was broken and was put in plaster for seven months! The whole experience was so unnecessary, fucking annoying, frustrating, humiliating and depressing, as no one had bothered to listen and understand what was happening. After all, the individual knows their own body better than anyone else. Taking time to understand and listen to an individual is really important and can aid recovery. I will never let being a spastic stop me! I will never let CP stop me either! Whichever way you look at it, to me,

I'm a spastic, and it's very liberating.

Over the years, I have pushed my body to extreme limits in order to maximise my independence, often forgetting about my cerebral palsy... It has to come with me, I don't go with it! I often ask myself if this is good or bad? I don't know the answer, but I live my life as able as possible in a spastic body and am determined not to give up.

And finally…

Oh Sal,
I want you to understand who the real me is
I want to educate and change and challenge people's perception.
I want people to see Kerry like you see Kerry
I want to be witty, funny, chatty and "boring"
Just like me really.
I want people to learn the real Kerry
The one behind the spastic body
I want to make people laugh, cry and question themselves.
I don't want much really!
I just want people to see me like you see me
Kerry!

Dear Sally

Oh Sally, can't believe it's 30 years since I last saw you, still doesn't make sense.

I always remember the first day I met you, I always knew that you and I were meant to be best friends. We liked and talked about the same stuff, had the crazy 80s perm poodle hairstyle and dressed in outfits with big bows and shoulder pads. What were we thinking of?

You made me laugh so much, causing trouble wherever we went. We went everywhere together, like terrible twins, inseparable! We learnt a lot together, but the one thing I didn't understand was your Cystic Fibrosis. Perhaps I didn't want to believe that one day you wouldn't be here or didn't want you to be in so much pain. I should have known deep down you wouldn't be here forever, as I knew your two sisters Jane and Janet passed away at a young age. Even the last days of your life I was in denial.

I held your hand and stroked your hair in hospital, praying for a miracle, right up until two days before you died. It was surreal, I couldn't believe you had gone. Those were the darkest days, especially when you're struggling with everything else as well. I honestly thought it was my time next... It felt so unfair that we wouldn't be getting into trouble ever again! I was only 14 and had lost you forever. A few days after my hospital visit you peacefully became my Guardian Angel in the sky watching over me.

I was determined to attend your funeral. I was as nervous as anything as I had never been to a funeral before. I had to laugh though when I saw my bouquet lying amongst the rest. They had spelt my name wrong. A nursery nurse from school crouched down on her hands and knees to put it right. It made everyone chuckle.

I kept my promise to you by keeping in touch with your devoted mum and dad every Christmas and birthday. We always remember what a massive part you played in our lives. Even now in my 40s, with a loving husband and two amazing children, I will always remember you and the bond that we shared.

Goodnight My Angel xxx

THE ABLE BODIES WRITE BACK!

By **ELAINE MASON**, May 2019

I got to know Kerry as a child growing up on the same housing estate in Wellingborough, Northants. Kerry lived in the next street but was a friendly face within the community. She has always been very independent even with her disability. We shared many experiences, lost touch but recently made contact again. It's as if we have always been there for each other.

At first Kerry would get a child from the street to knock on the front door as she couldn't get down the drive in her wheelchair. However, when she learnt to drive, Kerry drove past the house and bibbed her car horn several times, making me aware she was outside the house!

I was invited to join her and her parents on holiday in Great Yarmouth when we stayed at a bungalow on the outskirts. We spent many nights in the amusement arcades playing bingo or 2p machines. During the day we would go off and explore. We had our Tarot readings done, portraits drawn, went to see Jim Davidson at the Pier Theatre and afterwards went into his nightclub. One particular night we were heading back to the bungalow when we fancied some chips. But, as Kerry was desperate for the toilet, we went on ahead where the kerb was misjudged and Kerry ended up on the floor as she had tipped out of her chair. We laughed so much it didn't help Kerry as she was now dying for the toilet.

I helped Kerry complete her dissertation. I used to navigate our way to addresses that Kerry had recorded, some correct and some which I had a good guess at deciphering. When Kerry used to drive us to our destination, we have been up the wrong way of a one-way street, round the roundabout several times and got lost many a time. Many times we ended up crying with laughter due to her driving!

When we were old enough we used to go out on a Saturday night, mainly in Wellingborough itself. On returning to her flat, I would sleep on the floor with her two cats, Tia and Simba - anybody who knows me is aware that I'm not a cat person, Kerry used to find this funny when they tried to get in my sleeping bag!

By KEVAN THOMPSON

When Kerry asked me to write something for her book I asked, 'What would you like me to write?' The reply was typically Kerry, 'Oh, I dunno, anything. Write about what I was like at school.' How long ago was that? I was shocked to learn that more than thirty years had passed since I first met Kerry, which meant it was also more than thirty years since I had taught her. Despite the number of years we have kept in touch either through mutual friends, the odd celebration event or direct contact. We have over the years fell out of touch and then fell in touch. One way or another we have managed to follow each other's lives as we grew up, grew apart and then re- collided.

Throughout all this time she has remained a constant in the past of my career, someone I have recalled and shared with colleagues, friends and family.

I couldn't tell you when I first met Kerry but it was most likely in the corridor outside of the Physio room. Meeting her was when I was hit by a spider walking stick. As I walked past her and I said hello and she replied, 'Hi Sir,' and with her usual response of spasmodic reaction raised the stick involuntarily which just missed taking my head off my shoulders. She uttered the response 'Sorry' with a cheeky grin.

During those first few months my encounters were usually in the corridor trying to avoid being hit with flailing spider walkers or being run over as she attempted to master the use of a wheelchair. Despite nearly causing me actual bodily harm most exchanges were friendly and ended without major injury. Little was I to know that the young teenager who almost succeeded in squashing my toes or nearly giving me a black eye with her now familiar spasmodic movements would become a friend almost 30 years on and someone who I am immensely privileged to know. She is also for those who don't know her someone that once you have met you will never forget her, she certainly liked 'making people feel uncomfortable.' (Slogan from an advertising campaign Kerry took part in to raise awareness of disability)

My first lessons with Kerry were called 'Life Skills' but in reality they were Drama lessons which she relished in. During these lessons Kerry was able to practice skills in speaking and listening, debating real life issues including some very personal subjects. It was during one of these lessons that Kerry first asked me why we were referred to as a disabled school for children since a large number were young adults. She also went on to point out that the doors and toilets weren't disabled otherwise they would be unusable so why refer to them as disabled 'after all they weren't broken.' She would often make jokes about disabled people especially those with Cerebral Palsy, often commenting 'I'm one so I can say it.' She soon developed a reputation for challenging others and on more than one occasion landed herself in hot water with staff including the headteacher.

As Kerry progressed and grew in both age and confidence (hopefully helped through my teaching) she would use the drama lessons to challenge views. One of the issues she often loved to challenge was personal relationships and disabled people or as she would perhaps refer to it now 'Having sex.' This area was such a taboo subject but Kerry wanted more answers than simple facts; she wanted to challenge why it was seemingly wrong for disabled people to have intimate or sexual relationships.

One event which allowed her to present this to an audience came through a play we had, as a group written together called ‘Boy meets girl’. The story of how an able-bodied boy falls in love with a disabled girl despite the barriers put in place by her parents and the attitudes of others. After several weeks of rehearsals we put on the play to a mixed audience of students and parents followed by questions and answers. At the end of the play the final scene required Kerry to stand up out of her wheelchair and to be held in the arms of her on stage boyfriend. The play was a hit, even appearing in part on a local radio station, the final scene was greeted with gasps and comments such as ‘Wow, I didn’t know she could stand’ ‘Look they actually love each other’ and ‘Look they are holding each other.’ The question and answer session which followed was generally good humoured but took a serious turn when one parent became very cross that we had produced a play about such things as relationships, love and sex. Afterwards I recall Kerry’s response being along the lines of ‘Well that got them thinking’ along with the familiar cheeky grin.

At school Kerry was developing a reputation of a campaigner for disabled young people. Her frustration would show when other students seemed to accept their lot and would not join her crusade. With encouragement from other staff especially her English Teacher she successfully campaigned for a school uniform, which as she saw it would make her school the same as other high schools. She went on to challenge the local shopping centre about the lack of access for wheelchairs and a high street bank where a newly installed cash machine was up two steps and inaccessible for almost anyone with mobility problems.

As Kerry continued to develop into a young adult who enjoyed challenging ideas and making others feel uncomfortable, I like to think that the beginning of her gaining the confidence and skills to communicate those ideas started in those early lessons together. At a later stage when she got to university she was cast to take part in the TV movie Skallagrigg with a host of other well-known performers including Bernard Hill and Ian Dury. I first knew of this when a newspaper clipping arrived in the post from a former colleague. I cannot begin to express how proud I was when I found out, watching the movie I could see the Kerry I had come to know during those drama lessons, recognising some of the antics we had shared and I had been able to witness long before they made it onto the big screen.

Kerry probably is not aware but I used that movie several times as part of staff training sessions for years, we were apart but she very much remained a part of my career.

Of the many lessons I found myself teaching Kerry in, it was the less formal events which remain most vivid in my memory.

These include completing a Duke of Edinburgh Award Expedition and school residential visits. One of my roles in school was to work with a group of young people to develop a more vocational approach to learning. Part of this involved setting up a D of E group for young people with as they were then referred to 'Special Needs'. The activities in the main were school based and fairly straight forward. The challenge however would be the expedition part of the award. Within the group of students who were doing the D of E scheme were four students in wheelchairs and one severely visually impaired student, Kerry was part of this group.

Just to make life even more difficult the group with Kerry's enthusiasm decided that they should opt for a real challenge, if able-bodied people could climb hills why couldn't they? It was decided that climbing the likes of Snowdon or Scafell was out of the question largely because the Head would not sanction the visit. However the Long Mynd in Shropshire was fairly low level and had a road running almost the full length of the ridge. So 'all' we had to do was to get to the top and they could be transported back by minibus. What you have to bear in mind was that the walk was classified as an easy 6 miles and would take the average walker about two hours to complete, we had four manual wheelchairs and stiles to negotiate. Kerry was determined that she would complete this walk in or out of her wheelchair. The start of the walk began in a location called Ashes Hollow, a gentle gradient with gates which could be opened and a path seemingly accessible for wheelchairs.

To cut a long story short we ended up hauling, man handling, piggy back carrying and pushing both students and wheelchairs over about two thirds of the path, through gates and over stiles. For a large part Kerry walked with two staff on each side to support her. As we slowly trudged our way up the hillside at one point she turned towards me and said,

'My Physio told me that each step I take is the same as using 300 words.' I looked at her and after a short pause she then added,' So I want you to know sir that after doing this walk you have used up my words…so that's me buggered for my GCSEs.' Needless to say we did complete the walk, it took over eight hours and a lot of blood sweat and tears not to mention swearing which Kerry was more than capable of using.

Two other visits which I recall saw the Kerry we know now as she started challenging others and experienced prejudice close up. The first involved a visit to Carding Mill Valley, Shropshire as part of a longer visit to the area. The day was warm, the sky was blue, in fact a perfect day for a picnic so that's what we did. We found a suitable spot and those students in wheelchairs were asked if they wanted to sit on the grass. All including Kerry said yes. So over a period of about 20 minutes we assisted each student to move onto the grass. As the picnic progressed with sandwiches cakes and drinks (non-alcoholic) we were all sitting in a round having a chat and generally telling jokes, talking about this and that. Several people walked past, a few friendly ones said hello and waved. One particularly mature lady walked up to the group and towering over them all looked at each in turn then turned to myself and asked 'Are they enjoying themselves?'. This was like a red rag to a bull, Kerry, pulling herself up onto her knees beckoned the lady closer.

When she got to within arm's reach Kerry promptly grabbed her by the arm and pulled her closer. When their noses were almost touching she said in the loudest but most polite voice she could muster 'Yes and I take bloody sugar'.

On the same residential we also visited Llangollen to see the international Music Festival. I cannot remember if I was actually there or if this was reported back in the evening but the story goes something like this. Kerry was in her wheelchair along with another student also in a wheelchair being pushed along the main street in Llangollen, they passed a small craft style shop and Kerry asked if they could go inside. Turning into the shop doorway the owner greeted them, pointing at Kerry and the other student saying to the accompanying staff 'They can't come in here!' The fact that the owner had been so rude but had also directed his comments to the staff instead of the students just incensed Kerry. Her response was swift as she turned to both staff members and commented 'You can leave us here' so they did. Kerry and her friend then blocked the doorway to the shop and despite the owners protests they refused to move. After about 15 minutes the staff members returned upon which Kerry said they were ready to move on.

The owner was still complaining about customers not being able to get in or out of his shop, Kerry commented 'Serves him right next time he will take notice of people in wheelchairs!'

During the time I was teaching Kerry our first daughter was born. My wife brought our new daughter into school a few weeks following her birth as part of a child development activity. Kerry asked if she could hold our daughter. What do you do?

Here is a young girl with Cerebral Palsy who has a habit of suddenly going into spasm. If we handed her our daughter and she suddenly went into spasm we ran the risk of her throwing her onto the floor or at worse flipping her over her head. She asked several times wanting to hold her, so my wife carefully handed over our new baby, placing her into Kerry's arms, making sure she was safe and stepped back. To our surprise Kerry held our daughter for what seemed a lifetime and not once did she go into spasm and then assisted with both feeding and changing. We were so pleased to have been able to let Kerry hold our daughter and to trust her. We learned much later that when Kerry became pregnant with her own children and then holding them the result was the same as her spasms became much less.

When our second daughter was born the name we gave her was the same as Kerry's very closest friend who had recently died. This had quite an impact upon Kerry with her asking if we had named our daughter after her friend, I don't think we ever actually answered her question. Just for the record and to set things straight, 'Yes Kerry our daughter is named after your best friend.'

In recalling these times so many others re-emerge reminding me of other students. However one memory I have made both me and my then headteacher grin from ear to ear with what happened. I had moved to another school, my new school held a special prize giving event each year. We wanted a special guest to present the prizes, Kerry had completed her work on Skallagrigg and had just completed her university degree. She was not only a success but something of a celebrity. So we invited her and she agreed to come on the condition that she could do a workshop talking with our older students about facing challenges. Why not we thought and what a great role model, Kerry attended the prize giving on the agreed date and everything went really well until the workshop.

All the school leavers were invited along with various staff to the workshop which progressed well with students and staff firing questions towards Kerry. She answered them all with skill however one staff member then suggested that Kerry was giving our students false hopes and ambitions which they would not be able to achieve. Kerry promptly turned on the staff member and after a heated verbal exchange in which Kerry argued that they should still be encouraged to try, she finished with 'Just because I'm in a wheelchair it doesn't mean I'm thick!' Afterwards Kerry was describing what had happened to myself and the head, it took all our strength not to burst out laughing and punch the air.

I have been kept up to date with Kerry's exploits from former colleagues, friends and students over the years and still find it incredibly hard to believe who she has become. I have to keep pinching myself to remind me that she is now a mature woman, wife, mother and friend. In those first days of avoiding being hit by a spider walking stick one of the images I have is her cheeky grin and ability to always remain positive despite the twists and turns she has had to overcome to become the unique person she is. Her tenacity and determination continues and I hope never wanes. It came out of the blue when she asked me if I would write something for her story. It has perhaps taken longer than it should have but it has been good to recall some of the antics we got up too. The Kerry I know, someone who is fiercely independent, stands up against prejudice and someone who wants to be recognised first and foremost as a person and mum not because of her disability, I feel proud to have been allowed to be part of her world.

Fond memories and good times. Kev.

By **Helen Blakeman**, March 2018

In 2002 I followed up a referral for professional assistance from a young woman called Kerry Noble. Kerry had moved into the area I covered from Northampton with her two cats. The block of flats was far from ideal, with a block door, narrow corridor and front door in a corner. This was to be a long road we would work at together, to make her environment more suitable.

As circumstances changed so we would do a bit more. A rapport was built up between us through Kerry's struggles. The first thing on a visit was always to have a big hug and sometimes a few tears, but that was never dwelt on. On bad days I have had workmen who have visited to see how we could solve a problem. As big as they were they'd be in tears, not knowing how Kerry could get through some days, but she always did!

Kerry was and still is a very determined individual who knew what she wanted from life and was only hampered by her environment. Plus the fact that few professionals really understand fully how cerebral palsy affects individuals which Kerry finds extremely frustrating. Kerry has some very good supportive friends. The difficult times in some ways made her stronger and more determined to succeed in everything she does.

Educating students at Burleigh College on disability gave Kerry a purpose in life and I joined her several times to give students information on taking up a career working as a health professional. I got the feeling, on my visits to her classes that she got on very well with the students and I am sure the students admired her. Kerry used to be able to walk a few steps, but following a fall from her wheelchair she sustained injuries, which saw her in hospital for some time. This was a very bad time for Kerry as no one seemed to understand how her cerebral palsy affected decisions on treatment and her everyday living.

The one good thing that came out of her hospital stay was that at that time there was an older woman in the next bed and her son used to visit and also chat to Kerry. Then Maureen was discharged from hospital and Kerry was upset for her leaving but also felt she had lost the friendship of the women's son. To Kerry's surprise the young man, we now know as Chris, came and visited Kerry and the relationship grew and continued after being discharged from hospital.

In 2004 Kerry was desperate for a new wheelchair, so she decided to fund raise to enable her to obtain a suitable wheelchair. Kerry decided to do a parachute jump, which I felt, took a great deal of courage. I took a day off work to go and support her. We watched as she was lifted into the plane and took off. The person she was doing the tandem jump with kept her in the sky for a long time and on the floor we felt she would never land but she did. What an achievement.

That wasn't all! Next day Kerry took part in a fitness challenge with more than 30 people at Charnwood Leisure Centre, who hosted a treadmill challenge to assist with raising funds for her wheelchair. Kerry's friends wanted to help as they admired her efforts at exercising at the gym with an aim to fulfil her dream of being able to take a few steps down the aisle for her wedding later that year. Following the challenges we all met and had drinks at the golf club. This was a very proud day for me after all the hard work and determination Kerry had put in.

Chris had a rough time following the death of his mother but Kerry never gave up on him and they made plans to get married in Las Vegas. I wasn't able to attend although I would have loved to but watched the wedding live on a special link and was very proud to see Kerry standing with some support. I stayed as Kerry's occupational therapist and supported her through the next few years including when she became pregnant and had her first child Dylan.

I admired how Kerry, however difficult and painful life was, never gave up her determination to overcome every problem and, with assistance, looked after Dylan which was certainly a daily challenge. Eventually the flat was too small and a house was found for Kerry Chris and Dylan. It was altered in stages, and although far from perfect was much better than the flat.

I took early retirement but still visited Kerry, who will always be part of my life. Kerry had a brother for Dylan and both children are a credit to Kerry and Chris. Kerry was determined they would grow up as normal children and never become carers for her. They are wonderful well behaved children.

Kerry, Chris, Dilly and Charlie are a wonderful happy family, and I am very proud to be part of their lives.

Helen Blakeman

By **Jan and Perry Hall**, April 2018

I think that I have known Kerry for over fifteen years. I first met her when she was inspiring and supporting children at the special school, where I worked. She was then, as now, a positive force of nature and role model. When she asked me to contribute to her book I was honoured but also very perturbed. But you don't say 'no' to Kerry! What to write? A number of questions kept jumping into my head.

How much can I share with the reader? Not having read her manuscript, I wonder if her writing style mirrors the outrageously funny (and often politically incorrect) conversations that I have had with her over the years or has she adopted a more 'academic' and studious tone? Has she told anecdotes, such as the time that my husband accompanied her to an event, only for another man (who obviously thought that they were an item) to pass her his phone number as they left? (N.B. I must stress that this was before she was married!) Has she mentioned her ability to drink me under the table (albeit through a straw) and the 'Bailey's Effect'? Has she outlined her method of getting higher marks in pub quizzes or the way that she managed to get overtime payments for the crew when filming Skallagrigg? You would need to ask her, in person, about these! My lips are sealed!

Still not having seen what you have just read, I only hope that her larger than life character, warmth and humour shines through on every page. I am sure that it will.

In the, very popular, musical Wicked by Stephen Schwartz, there is a song called Defying Gravity in which the leading lady sings 'No Wizard that there is or was, is ever gonna bring me down!' In my opinion, this could be Kerry's anthem. The 'Wizard' in the musical, as in the Wizard of Oz, is a man who convinces his citizens to believe the untrue. The 'Wizard', in Kerry's case might be the people and organisations that have led many to believe, over the years, that people like Kerry need to settle for less in life due to 'additional' needs. It could, indeed, be argued that we all have additional needs because we are all individual and unique and none of us has exactly the same needs as everyone else. It could also be suggested that the 'Wizard', in Kerry's case, might be individuals who, due to a lack of understanding and/or empathy, have placed barriers in her way such as the traffic warden who, having watched her park her adapted car, get her electric wheelchair from the roof and travel away in it, then gave her a ticket because her disability pass was upside down!

It is true, however, that Kerry does not let any of this 'bring her down'. She will not let anyone ignore her and speak to the person with her as if she is not there or cannot communicate (as happened to us once at the theatre when Kerry informed the man who asked me if I had brought her that she had, in fact, brought me)! She 'defies gravity' daily and has been doing so for all the years that I have known her, long before the more current focus on inclusion. She is inspirational as she gives talks to others; drives to venues (usually at top speed, which I found terrifying on my first outing with her); whips to the shops in the rain; is mum to her wonderful family; gets involved as a governor or parent in education; parties hard; tells very entertaining stories; the list is endless. In fact, she does everything and more than somebody who has not got a condition that must, let's face it, be both painful and frightening at times. She grabs life by the scruff of the neck; gets what she wants and when she wants it. Good for her! Her husband, Chris, should also get a special mention here (although I suspect that she will edit this out)!

I cannot wait to read what she has to say and hope that her words vanquish the 'Wizard' in people who do not look beyond a 'disability' and inspires both those who might perceive barriers facing them and those who are intrigued by the life- stories of others.

I only hope that there is enough ink in the printer for the amount of asterisks that might need to be inserted because of her aforementioned 'colourful' language or that her editor has a sharp and thick pencil!

Jan Hall

By **Jane Howard-White**

Kerry Coe, or Kerry Noble, as she was when I first met her in the year 2000 – what to say about this inspiring, brave, determined, stubborn, funny woman, colleague, friend and mother?

I work for a tiny local charity in Bedford supporting people whose lives have been affected by cerebral palsy and associated disabilities. One day back in 2000 I was called by Kerry. It took me a while to tune into Kerry's voice as her CP does have an effect on her speech and after she patiently repeated herself to me I began to understand and ask for repetitions less.

It turned out that Kerry wanted to apply for a Millennium Volunteer place, which were being funded across the country. Kerry had an idea for a project that she would like to deliver and needed an organisation that could support the delivery of the project and provide a Mentor (or a mental as Kerry came to introduce me as)

I agreed to meet Kerry at her home in Wellingborough and

her engaging personality, drive and determination to live life to the full and the profile photo on her phone that said 'Tart on Wheels' had me hooked in.

Kerry soon became a much loved part of the BDCPS 'family' She created a project delivering disability awareness the Kerry Noble way. Honest and no holds barred. The project was called Disability, It doesn't have to make a difference and, of course, this is how Kerry has lived her life in the main.

Kerry drove a car with an adaptation to carry her chair. She travelled the length and breadth of Bedfordshire delivering tailor-made awareness sessions to young people in their schools, social groups etc. from an age range of four to 25 and also did several special school and specialist charity staff team meetings. Even after she gave up her car and moved away to live in Loughborough, she would catch the train fully loaded with a massive suitcase full of equipment that was as big as her and juggled her handbag and phone on her lap. Kerry kept this going for a number of years and many Bedfordshire young people have had their lives enriched by the very personal and real insight that people are people and disability does not have to make a difference.

This millennium project was a huge success and Kerry was nominated for The Volunteer of The Year Award. She, of course, was shortlisted and won the award in her category after a night in a plush London Hotel and a swanky presentations event.

As a pregnant woman Kerry agreed to come along and star in a training video where we filmed lots of potential bad care practice. She endured moving and handling and humiliating experiences in a chip shop and other environments. All this to help staff and volunteers to think and question their practice and better understand and enable those they serve. Even now Kerry drags the family over to Bedford so that she can support the charity with its annual staff and volunteer training week.

Kerry always strived to live an 'ordinary' life but I think it's fair to say given the extent of her CP she has certainly lived an extraordinary one.

Kerry became a close friend and I love her dearly. She is amazing and throws herself into anything that she wants to do. From the moment I met her and across the years I stand in awe of her.

Jane Howard-White

By **Megan Bruce**, May 2019

I first met Kerry when she came into my office to introduce herself. I had recently become her social worker after she had a really rough experience with both social services and the NHS. I was immediately overwhelmed by her determination and courage, I was in awe of her.

Through my time spent working with Kerry there were some serious life changing decisions that had to be made due to the awful cuts the councils are facing. She accepted them with dignity and worked hard to remain the fierce, independent women she is. It was a pleasure getting to know her and Chris and we remain friends long since finishing work together. I feel proud to be able to call her a friend and to hear about her latest adventures. May she long continue to throw herself off mountains!

Megan Bruce

By **Simone Harvey**, June 2018

'Hi, it's Kerry, I've heard you're interested in working with me? What days and hours are you looking for? I'm just in hospital in labour …'

This was my first ever dealing with Kerry, a text message while she was in labour with her first child! Little did I know at that time that message sums Kerry up in one! Nothing will get in the way of her arranging and organising things in her life, not even childbirth!

A week or so later I met Kerry, Chris and their new baby for an interview for the support worker position she had available. We hit it off straight away and I started supporting Kerry a few weeks later. Eight years on and I'm still here. I get Kerry; I know when to back away or keep my mouth shut and nose out which I know is very important to her and her independence. We've been through a lot together over the years, Botox, tattoos, very nearly child birth with her second child. Luckily I managed to get her into the ambulance with only minutes to spare!

I've witnessed Kerry at her absolute best and at rock bottom. Amazingly she carries on regardless. Nothing stands in her way, which I admire deeply. She has a wonderful family and two beautiful children who are a real credit to both her and Chris. Seven years into my support role with Kerry I have now become part of her family as she has mine and I'm thankful for all the opportunities she has given to me (apart from asking me to do a skydive with her, which I refused!).

I plan on being part of this family for many years to come.

Simone Harvey

By **Steve Hackney**

I met Kerry through my then girlfriend and her parents in Vicarage Farm Social Club. I was 18 and Kerry was 12 and lived next door.

The first thing I remember was Kerry coming downstairs on her arse, giggling and making fun of the situation. This was true Kerry style – it was Kerry through and through. She used to get around on her arse and also sit on the floor in front of the settee. When Kerry was 16, she used her wheelchair to get around town including The Arndale shopping centre. You knew Kerry was on her way as all you could hear was the horn on her wheelchair and Kerry laughing. At this point there were no electric doors and Kerry campaigned so she could get access to the shopping centre They are still there today.

When Kerry decided to learn how to drive and pass her test, she needed to raise money to convert a car to her needs. So Sandra approached the club to do a fund-raising night to help Kerry. She got her car and typical of Kerry a car sticker that said spastic in control, But the Unemployed Workers

Association asked Kerry to remove it.

Kerry's car was converted to hand controls. Well, if you ever get the chance to try this you should – I did and it's not as easy as it looks. The car made me look like a learner and Kerry the professional at a time when I drove trucks for a living. The car had a top box that carried Kerry's wheelchair.

When Kerry was 18 and was old enough to go into the pubs, we went on nights out in town. She also had weekends with the girls.

When Kerry got a place at university, off she went on her own in her little car and friends went to visit her there. She passed her degree with the hard work and determination she has shown her whole life.

This is where life gave us different paths to follow and Kerry and I lost contact. After university, Kerry got her own flat and I went to visit her. After this I used to pop up from Wellingborough to see her. Every time Kerry was in hospital I used to visit her. One time she told me about Chris, a man she had met there. On this particular visit Kerry was in traction.

When Kerry came out of hospital, she and Chris stayed in contact and became partners. A few years later, Kerry announced that she and Chris were getting married in the White Chapel in Las Vegas. Their wedding video was online and Kerry gave me a link so I could watch it . A few weeks later they had a wedding reception.

Chris was quite the worse for wear at the reception and Kerry's parents asked me to look after her and what I thought of their marriage. I replied that they were consenting adults and good luck to both of them.

They had been married for four years when Kerry announced she was pregnant. Then around six months later Dylan-Grace arrived. 4 months later she was pregnant again but sadly this one became a butterfly and flew away into the sky. A year later on Kerry asked me to be around for Dylan whilst she was in hospital to have another baby. I stayed in Kerry's house, but this was when I chose quite by accident to lock myself out of the car and had to ring Chris to get Dylan from nursery and let me in the house.

Not only this, imagine this if you can: when I took Dylan to see Mum, Dad and little brother Charlie James. Dylan needed a baby change and I had put the new baby's nappy on an 18-month-old. Kerry found this highly amusing.

It was during this visit when Kerry and Chris bestowed on me the honour of being Charlie's godfather, to which I agreed. I am now a regular visitor to Kerry and her family with my family.

Steve Hackney

By **Leah Stirrat**

I first met Kerry in the autumn of 1986. When I started teaching at a "Special school" for children with "physical disabilities". I had already taught in various secondary schools and had trained as primary school teacher. Along the way, I had encountered a range of students with diverse needs and abilities.

During my first year, Kerry was not in one of my teaching groups, but whenever I met her in a corridor she gave me her trademark "big smile" and cheerily greeted me. I was on a steep learning curve finding out and understanding about Cerebral Palsy and I quickly understood that there are as many variations in CP as there are humans on the planet.

Kerry was a bright child with an enthusiasm for learning, but also willing to try and see how little work she could get away with .....

I realised that Kerry could achieve far more than some people gave her credit for, so I set the bar high and raised her self-expectations. She could achieve GCSEs and she did. She could go to college and she did. She would get to university and she did. Attending her graduation was one of the proudest moments in my life.

I know that life hasn't always been easy for Kerry but she has achieved so much.....I am proud to know her and be her friend.

Over the years I have been part of her growing up and all the different stages of her life. Marriage, Motherhood, holidays, family times and celebrations. All of which have been special and important. Kerry and her family have become part of our family ....she grew up with our children and now her children are growing up with our grandchildren. If people ask me who Kerry is .... I say she is my "adopted" daughter and her children ....two more grandchildren.

I sometimes think Kerry has achieved so much because of her CP and it has made her the person she is: feisty, hardworking, caring, compassionate, understanding, organised, loving, and a really good lifetime friend.

Leah Stirrat

By **Fiona Dunne**

I first met Kerry when we were teenagers at Tile Hill College in Coventry; it's shocking thinking about it now because that was 29 years ago! We've known each other that long!? We were in the same welfare and society class. Kerry, Janice (another close friend) and I hit it off as soon as we met each other.

I have memories of her living in her own flat at Hereward College and cooking for herself, Janice and me sometimes. That's how independent she was. We finally left college and went our separate ways, eventually losing contact. Years later I was thrilled when I found her again using social media!

How can I describe Kerry? She is this extremely strong woman who is intelligent, fiercely independent, extremely positive, assertive and very organised. I really look up to and admire her!! She is proof that having a disability doesn't have to stop an amazing woman such as Kerry living life to the full. (I hope you don't mind me saying this, Kerry).

But most of all Kerry is a really great friend. I've often thought that she would make a really good counsellor because she is a really good listener.

Fiona Dunne

By **Su Carroll**

Despite my lack of writing skills and my stereotypical Yorkshire bluntness, I was pleased to be asked to write a piece about Kerry. Kerry thinks highly of her friends and being chosen to appear in her life story proves she thinks of me as a true friend. She wears her heart on her sleeve and will always make it clear who she values and appreciates in her life.

We met at an amazing parent and baby group at the local Children's Centre. We were there with our daughters, she with her new-born and I with my six-month-old. I admired her from the start for the way she persevered with breastfeeding difficulties, coped with baby sleep problems and was eager to succeed as a mother.

As many parents do, I had my own concerns about being a good mother and was anxious I was doing it all wrong.

However, I could see how proud Kerry was of the new bundle of joy she had brought into the world and this helped to empower me. Maybe we could be alright at this new

motherhood lark and I wasn't doing so badly after all.
After the parent and baby group came to an end, we didn't see a lot of each other in those first years and weren't particularly close but when our paths did cross we were always pleased to see each other, offer each other advice and share the highs and lows of caring for our daughters.

We were both happy to hear that the other was pregnant with a second child. Both babies were boys and born within a couple of months of each other. Now, with two children of similar ages, we saw much more of each other and became close friends.

Kerry became the host of her famous (amongst those in the know) 'Cowboy Pie' parties, in which she hosts several children and friends, plies them with drinks, food, party games, treats and prizes, ensuring everyone feels welcome and happy. The children play and bond together while the adults attempt to chat and catch-up amongst the lively commotion.

Over the years I have gradually learned more about Kerry and the interesting life she leads. I am pretty quiet so it is good to spend time with someone who likes to talk and she really likes to talk. She has starred in a film, been to Number 10, had an awkward interaction with a former Prime Minister and met her husband in unusual, fortuitous circumstances. She also has a steadily increasing number of self-designed tattoos; is possibly the most organised person I have ever met (birthday parties and holidays are planned down to the smallest detail several months in advance) and a serial skydiver.

I would never have the nerve to jump out of an aeroplane and, thinking about it, neither would the majority of people. Kerry however is not like the majority of people, she is very, very determined and when she decides she wants to do something, she will do her best to make sure it happens. As an able-bodied person I cannot begin to imagine her exhilaration and sense of freedom of flying through the air, at however many miles an hour, with only a parachute for safety.

Kerry has cerebral palsy, which means she is confined mostly to a wheelchair and has to rely on support workers for physical tasks. Even going to the toilet is something that she cannot accomplish without someone being there to assist (apart from that time she was desperate for a wee after downing a bottle of wine, but that's another story!).

Over the years Kerry and her family have become a big part of our lives. They are there for us in lieu of geographically distant family – taking my children to various activities and events, inviting them for tea dates or sleepovers and showing fondness for them. Unlike my daughter who is completely bemused by it, I appreciate and understand her husband's dry sense of humour. Her daughter is an exceptional reader, thanks to her mother's commitment and perseverance, and she is polite, outgoing and a good friend to my daughter. Her son has been brought up an intelligent and happy boy and he and my son are great buddies.

I told my four-year-old son that I had been asked to write a piece for Kerry's book and asked what he thought I should say. His response was simply 'I love Kerry'.

Su Carroll

By **James Taylor-Coe**

Kerry, my evil step mum Kerry. This is what she calls herself to me, but in truth she is the absolute opposite.

I remember meeting Kerry for the first time at the hospital where my grandma was unfortunately in. I instantly took a liking to her, mainly because she gave me a box of chocolates, but also because I could see how happy she made my Dad as they joked and chuckled together in each other's company. Little did I know this woman was here to stay?

After our introduction over the coming months I got to know Kerry and would regularly bump into her around Loughborough. Always full of energy and happiness she would be on some sort of mission. This seems to be a trend over the years and once Kerry has an aim or goal, she will not slow down or stop until it is complete (even this autobiography!). Regularly using this drive to help worthy causes such as Small World nursery, she will rise to any challenge, even jumping out of a plane!

After watching Kerry change from a cat mother to an actual

mother you can see the change and her ever increasing energy levels. Dylan-Grace and Charlie-James will one day look back and see what an attentive and passionate Mum they have and will hopefully take on these qualities themselves.

From night clubbing in Ibiza to days out in London with my brother and sister we have had lots of good times and I look forward to many more to come.

James Taylor-Coe

AND FINALLY, FINALLY, IT'S THANKS FROM ME!

I really hope you decided to relax and enjoy my sense of humour around disability and the way I live with my life to the full as a spastic. I hope you appreciate my honesty and personality as it's taken a lot of charisma and determination to fight back from the social model of disability and stand up for my beliefs.

It's taken me a long time and a lot of soul searching to produce Spasm. It has always been my long-term aim since I was a teenager. As I grew up, I always felt different and no one understood an able mind in a spastic body, especially when you were born this way. I wanted to share my experiences and determination.

I would like to dedicate this book to my loyal and devoted husband Chris, without his full backing and support, I wouldn't be where I am today. Also, to our children, Dylan-Grace, Charlie-James and James, as well as our guiding star Charlie- Grace. I owe a great thank you to you all.

This book is to enable you to learn much more about Mummy's life and experiences and to remember never to give up even when times are hard and challenging. Always remember you can do anything you set your mind to.

I would like to thank several devoted special people in my life for their contributions in their own way, in my life as well as in this book and shared experiences and standing by my side through thick and thin throughout the years.

Thank you for believing in me and putting up with my stubborn, rebellious and determined ways. None of this would be possible without your love and support.

Thank you goes to:

- My husband, Chris Coe. You are my soul mate, you make everything possible, even when we don't see eye to eye. You've made my dream come true, you've believed in me and enabled Spasm to become a reality. Endless hours of typing and nagging. Thank you for putting up with my determined barriers and menopausal state of mind. You've always put up with me through thick and thin. You are my soul mate, you are my determination, you're the one who kicks my arse when I need it! I love you!

My children:

- o Dylan-Grace Coe (you might recognise this name from the front inside cover…)
- o Charlie-James Coe
- o Charlie-Grace Coe
- o James Taylor-Coe

Without you none of this would be possible. Thank you for seeing me for me. I love you all. Thank you Dilly for your own special words, they mean everything to me.

My extended family:

- o Leah & Ian Stirrat
- o Jan & Perry Hall
- o Helen Blakeman
- o Steve Hackney
- o Elaine Mason
- o Kevan Thompson
- o Bernard Hill

Thank you for supporting me throughout my life, being there in times of need and believing in me.

My friends:

- Jane Howard-White
- Su Carroll
- Emma Wing
- Fiona Dunne
- Thank you for many years of true friendship and seeing me for me.

Everyone who has made this book a reality:

- Michelle Catanach
- Wendy & John Dickinson from Enrych Charity
- Maddie Bailey from Enrych Charity
- John Brindley from Enrych Charity
- Enrych Charity
- Bren & Claire for reading Spasm
- Megan Bruce
- Jess Reed
- Liv Cornwell

Thank you for supporting me throughout this journey and producing Spasm, and being there throughout the good and bad times of what life throws at you. You have all helped enable me to fulfil this lifelong goal and create Spasm. You have all held your own individual input.

Current and past support workers who have lived to survive the experience. Especially thanks to Simone Harvey and Jackie Lewin for their dedication and commitment shown to me and my family over the last 9 years, without you it wouldn't be possible.

Last but not least, Millie Rice. Special thanks for enabling Spasm to come alive again after so long and reaching my goal to get it to the publisher on time before you embark on your new postgraduate job.

For more information on Cerebral Palsy and related conditions please visit:

www.cerebralpalsy.org/about-cerebral-palsy/definition

or Bedfordshire Scope:

https://www.scope.org.uk

www.ingramcontent.com/pod-product-compliance
Lightning Source LLC
LaVergne TN
LVHW050532160826
845677LV00011B/2008

9798552062522